Keto Diet Over 50

Simple Suggestions and 30-Minutes Low Carb Recipes to Easily Reach Ketosis and Get Back on Track With 28 Days Meal Plan Included.

Penny Craig

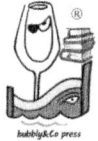

bubbly&Co press

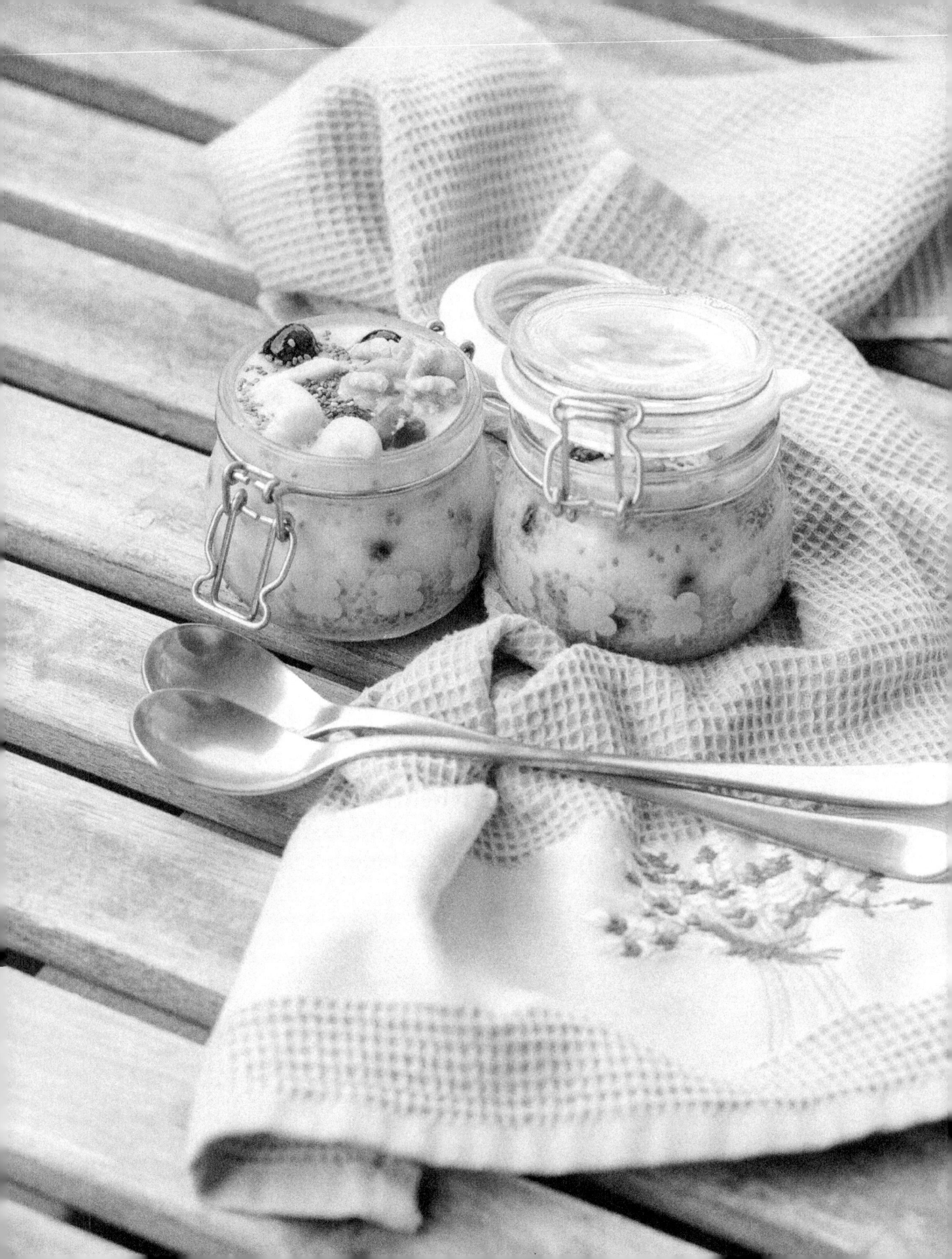

Copyright 2021 – Penny Craig
All rights reserved.

The content contained within this book may not be reproduced, duplicated, or transmitted without direct written permission from the author or the publisher. Under no circumstances will any blame or legal responsibility be held against the publisher, or author, for any damages, reparation, or monetary loss due to the information contained within this book. Either directly or indirectly.

Legal Notice:

This book is copyright protected. This book is only for personal use. You cannot amend, distribute, sell, use, quote or paraphrase any part, or the content within this book, without the consent of the author or publisher.

Disclaimer Notice:

Please note the information contained within this document is for educational and entertainment purposes only. All effort has been executed to present accurate, up to date, and reliable, complete information. No warranties of any kind are declared or implied. Readers acknowledge that the author is not engaging in the rendering of legal, financial, medical, or professional advice. The content within this book has been derived from various sources. Please consult a licensed professional before attempting any techniques outlined in this book.

By reading this document, the reader agrees that under no circumstances is the author responsible for any losses, direct or indirect, which are incurred because of the use of information contained within this document, including, but not limited to, errors, omissions, or inaccuracies.

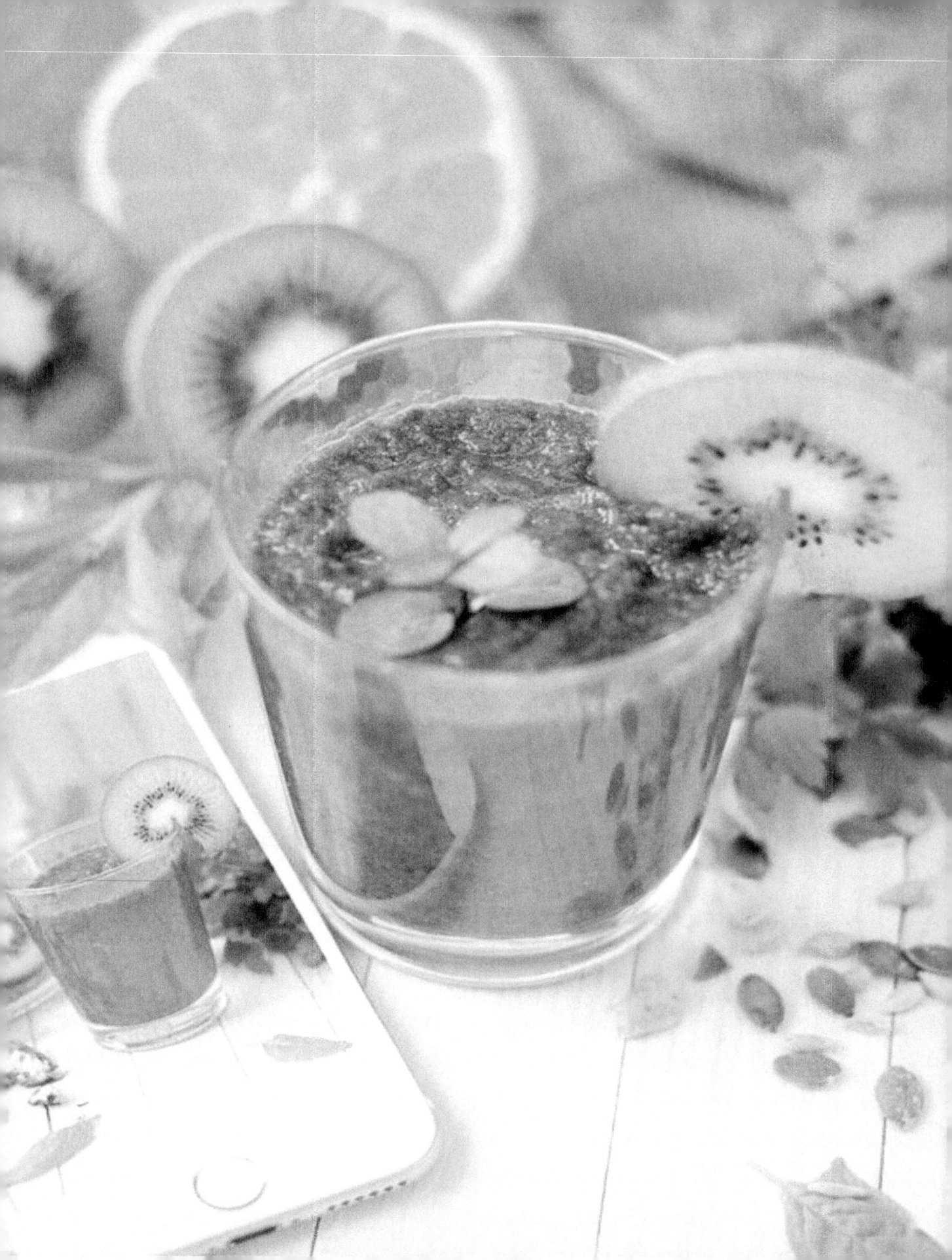

INTRO	7
PART 1	
1. SIMPLY KETO	11
2. MIND & BODY AT 50+	33
3. EQUIPMENT & TOOLS	53
PART 2	
4. KETOGENIC MEETS MEDITERRANEAN	63
5. NUTRITION, WORKOUT & REST AT 50+	71
6. TOP 55 KETO MED RECIPES	81
7. MEASUREMENT CONVERSION	155
8. 28 DAYS MEAL PLAN	157
CONCLUSION	161
AUTHOR OVERVIEW	164

Intro

The strive and goal of this guide is to deepen the concept behind the ketogenic diet, nutrition around 50 (before, during, and after), the symptoms of **keto flu**, and the overall benefits of the diet.

Currently, the ketogenic diet is a popular method of nutrition, revolving around strict adherence to the rules that the diet itself imposes, used for centuries, since ancient Greek times.

Historians have shown us that the Greeks were the first to report that the effects of certain diseases and disorders could be alleviated, if not cured completely, by following a particular and strict dietary routine.

One of the chronic syndromes they frequently treated with dietary restrictions was epilepsy, known then as "**having fits**." They noticed that people who suffered from epilepsy and followed the keogenic diet improved significantly.

The 20th century provided us with the first modern study of the effects of the keto diet on "**fits**", which later came to be known as **epilepsy**. Studying a group of patients, doctors discovered that they could limit the number of daily fits by having them follow, a low-calorie, low-carbohydrate, high-fat diet.

Since drugs did not yet exist at that time, the only help in the medical field, to improve the patient's health, was to harness the benefits of diet by combining them with daily physical activity.

Examining the results of the study further and trying to determine the reason for the success, the scientists found that the ketogenic diet induced the production of three different chemical compounds in the human body, that were water-soluble and were present only in the bodies of people who were starving or on a high-fat, low-carbohydrate diet.

Scientists christened these chemical bodies "ketone bodies" hence the term ketogenic diet or keto for short.

Early ketogenic diets were very different in the ratio of protein to fat consumed. Doctors had the idea of trying the diet on patients with epilepsy, allowing them to eat until completely full, provided their meals were high in fat, with a moderate amount of protein but low in carbohydrates.

The recommendation was that carbohydrate intake should not exceed 20 grams of the patient's total daily food intake.

This plan reduced the number of ailments, and even eliminated them, plus it produced other beneficial side effects: patients were able to sleep better for longer periods of time.

Vigilance and attention were dramatically increased, and children who were on the diet also showed improved behaviour.

This diet was widely used as a treatment for epilepsy until the mid-20th century, when drugs were developed to treat this chronic syndrome, taking a spoonful of syrup or swallowing a pill was much easier, than struggling and following such a restrictive diet.

However, it was difficult to stick to this diet as certain types of food was not easily available, refrigeration of goods was not yet widely available at this time, and many people did not have access to fresh dairy products such as milk, cheese, and eggs, especially those who lived in big cities.

Much of the population survived on a diet of vegetables grown in their home garden and these were the staple of their daily diet.

The keto diet intended as medical therapy was being used less and less, so much so that it was no longer taught in medical schools, consequently, becoming a mere historical record in medical books.

In the 1960s and 1970s, the Western population began to pay more attention to their personal looks and health; media grew during these years which contributed to the rise of international fashion trends.

The bikini was the swimsuit that all women wanted to wear. Fashion diets were also successful because they were advertised with the guarantee of rapid weight loss, achieving a beautiful body and lasting fitness.

During this period the keto diet was rediscovered and once again enjoyed great popularity, different versions were created by different experts who gave their names to the diet plans.

The keto diet reached it's highest point of popularity in the 1990s thanks to the news of a child whose fits were so serious that medication could not relieve them.

The little boy's parents desperately searched for a remedy that could reduce and cure their son's suffering, and so by studying the medical literature they learned that the keto diet was originally used to treat-control epilepsy.

The keto diet was an alternative way to try to treat their child's syndrome. Shortly after starting the keto diet, he stopped having serious fits that had plagued him since birth.

Deeply grateful and thankful they decided to publicize their story through a documentary, and again the keto diet came to the forefront as one of the best natural methods for curing chronic syndromes and superfluous weight loss. Many people undertook the keto diet and were pleased with the obvious and lasting results of an original therapy developed to treat epileptic seizures in adults and children.

The basis of the keto diet is the same as that of our ancestors, who were hunter-gatherers of any fruits and vegetables, which they supplemented with the meat they hunted. Our ancestors' diet was heavily based on meat and fat, with the occasional berries or carrots.

Many generations later, we have become more overweight because our lifestyles have become more sedentary, and our eating habits are unbalanced, concentrated on exaggerated consumption of carbohydrates, farinaceous foods, sweet, carbonated drinks, and industrial convenience foods.

So, what is it that makes the keto diet the perfect solution for weight loss and disease prevention? The root cause of all these wonderful side effects is known as **Ketosis.**

1. Simply Keto

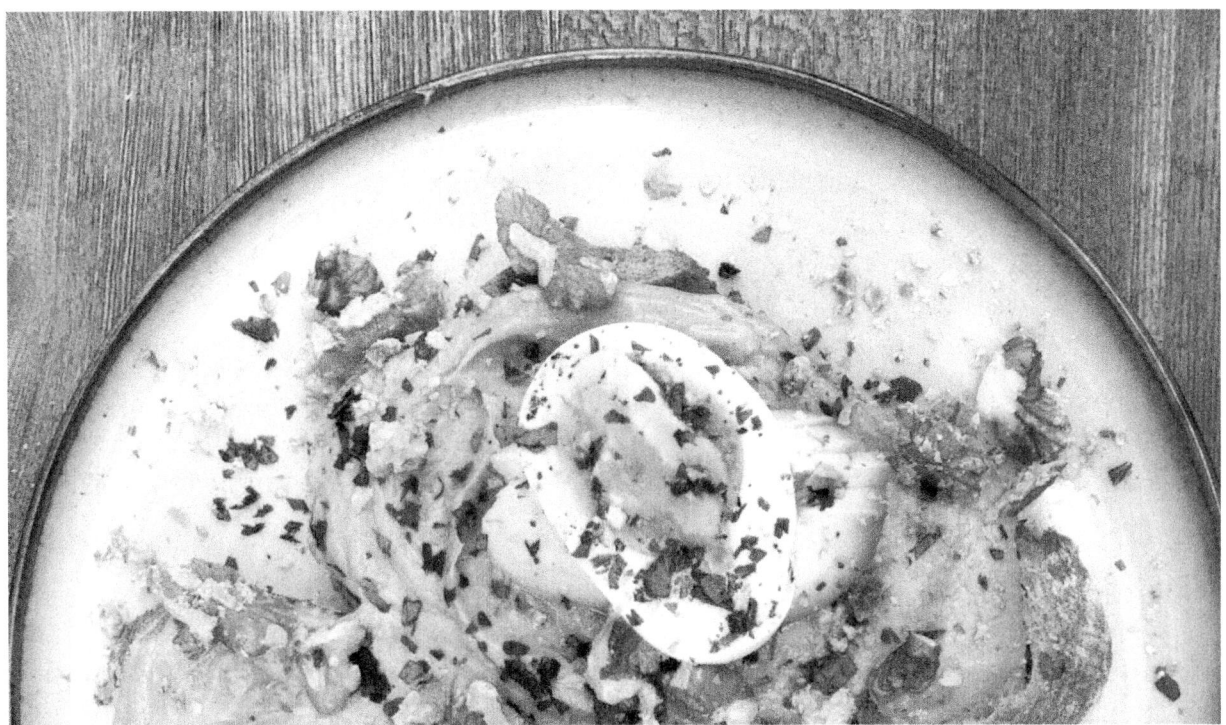

Keto What?

The ketogenic diet is an alimentary program that involves a low consumption of carbohydrates, a medium consumption of protein and a high consumption of fat. The positive implications of this diet are the reduction of body fat, simply because, thanks to this type of nutrition the metabolism is hacked, by doing so the human body then starts burning fat (ingested or stored) instead of glucose, as the primary source of daily energy.

The "Keto" diet reached world heights of popularity after the mid-1910s. Throughout the 21st century, people who followed keto with commitment, determination and training, this diet plan found a marked improvement in their overall health, improved muscle tone and regained well-being.

Keto How?

Keto is a very low-carb diet (minimum 20 grams per day).

Not per meal...yes...you read that right, but 20 grams per day.

It is not for the faint-hearted and lovers of pasta and bread...it is a nutritional method that requires complete dedication, but it amply repays sustained efforts.

It is not easy, especially in the beginning, and some people find it simply too restrictive or difficult to maintain. On the other hand, if you are trying to lose weight and generally improve your health ...Keto is definitely for you.

One of the most important nutrients to fuel our brains is glucose or sugar. When glucose levels are low, due to low carbohydrate intake, our bodies begin to burn fat and ketones as fuel instead of glucose.

Ketosis is the state in which the body produces ketones in the liver to use as energy. These ketones are produced from fat (the breakdown of fatty acids), with the help of protein (the synthesis of amino acids), the process usually begins when insulin levels are low, breaking down fats quickly to generate energy for the cells in the brain, muscles, and all other organs.

The brain is made up primarily of fat, and so the main problem with any diet that reduces carbohydrates is how to provide energy for the brain. Ketones are an ideal energy source because they have a low oxidation rate and because they are full of lipids (fats), they do not require much oxygen to fuel them.

Muscles can use ketones as fuel for proper function.

Through oxidative phosphorylation an energy-producing biochemical mechanism, using the molecule ATP(Adenosine-Tri-Phosphate), by separation of Phosphate from Adenosine by hydrolysis, energy used for all cellular processes in the human body is released.

What Is Ketosis?

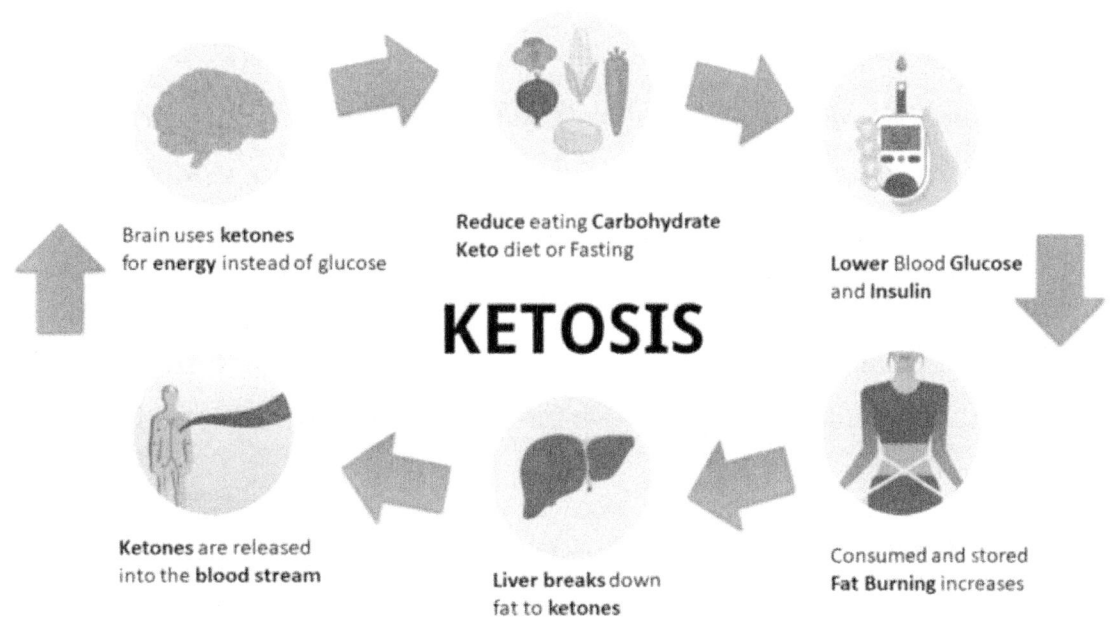

Ketosis is a metabolic state, in which part of the human body's energy supply comes from ketone bodies released from the liver into the bloodstream.

The goal of this eating plan is to burn fat and improve overall health; in fact, Keto is widely recognized as one of the most effective ways to feel lighter, motivated, vital and focused.

The first step to entering ketosis is to reduce your consumption of carbohydrates (glucose or starch) and added sugars. To make this diet work, you need to keep well-hydrated, consume fruits and vegetables indicated for their fiber content, and exercise daily.

If you follow the rules correctly, you will enter ketosis within 12-48 hours, at which point, your body will begin to use ketones (fat) as its primary energy source, in doing so you will notice a decrease in body fat stores resulting in weight loss.

Evidence of Ketosis

According to many studies, people who follow this diet have a much lower risk of developing chronic diseases, such as type 2 diabetes, heart disease, dementia, and general inflammation.

Keto diets allow for significant fat reduction due to its ability to stabilize blood sugar levels, however, this carefully followed eating plan, with the help of exercise, preserves long-term health and well-being by improving insulin sensitivity and lowering the risk of cardiovascular disease.

Athletes often use this dietary strategy to increase the availability of energy (in the form of ATP) for resistance-based exercise. They get a huge amount of energy from using fat as fuel, resulting in increased and improved athletic performance.

The keto diet is also an excellent alternative for those who do not find satisfaction by following other diets; this eating plan is favourable because it keeps them fuller for longer periods of time.

Testing of Ketosis

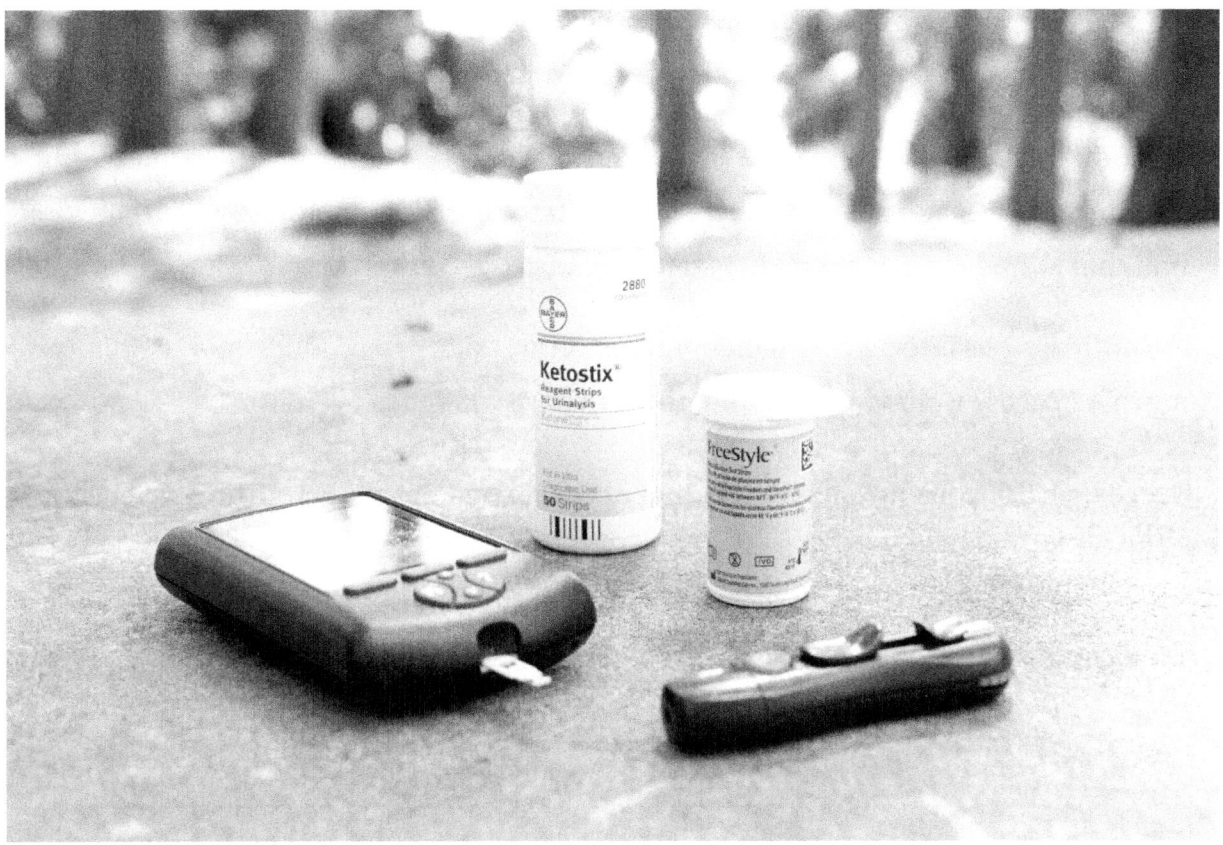

There are 3 methods to test the state of Ketosis in the human body:

- ➢ **breath test** measures the level of acetone
- ➢ **blood test** measures the level of beta-hydroxybutyrate
- ➢ **urine test** measures the level of acetone acetate

One of the easiest and cheapest ways to determine if the human body is in ketosis is to use urine test strips. You can buy them online or at any pharmacy, this simple test, ascertains the presence or absence of acetoacetate, a ketone body, confirming or denying with some approximation, the state of Ketosis.

Checking ketones at the beginning of the diet helps us ascertain the state of nutritional ketosis and thus confirm that we are burning fat instead of glucose. This check also allows us, a little at a time, to figure out what the amount of daily carbohydrates might be that allows us to maintain the state of ketosis, which is necessary to continue the diet.

Starting with 20 g of carbohydrates per day for 2-3 days, monitoring, then increasing to 30 g for 2-3 days and so on, with the goal of finding the very individual carbohydrate limit that allows us to maintain the state of ketosis.

The ultimate goal is to achieve metabolic flexibility, that is, to produce energy by burning fat when glucose is not available and using glucose when it is present.

The change from one metabolic state to the other should happen quite quickly, meaning, that if we fall out of ketosis state, it will no take as much time to re-enter as it did the first time. The process will be much faster, thus regaining the natural human ability to produce energy, for our daily needs, using fats.

Examples of Ketosis

The keto diet is used by athletes all over the world, from long-distance runners who consume less than 50 grams of carbohydrates a day to boxers, world champions, who consume 10 eggs every morning. It is important that you find what works best for you.

There are many variations of the ketogenic diet that have been created over time. Some are stricter than others and some have special requirements.

Keto Benefits

- Stabilizes insulin: Insulin is a hormone produced in the pancreas that is responsible for moving glucose in the blood and storing it as fat in the human body. Keto is a dietary method suitable for decreasing high insulin levels caused by ingesting too many refined carbohydrates (pasta, bread, starchy foods, etc.). By limiting carbohydrate consumption, the risk of insulin resistance antechamber to type 2 diabetes is reduced.
- Reduces Inflammation: inducing the body to use ketone bodies (fat) as fuel instead of glucose(carbohydrates) is found to have significant benefits for those suffering from inflammatory complications such as arthritis, autoimmune disorders, diabetes, chron's disease, this is because' decreasing glucose production reduces inflammatory states related to excess blood sugar.
- Reducing Emotional Hunger: Eating to satiety avoids the unregulated consumption of junk food and processed sweets, helping to decrease to the point of elimination, emotional eating, which is responsible for the onset of inflammation and chronic diseases.
- Fat Burning: If the goal is a way to teach the human body how to burn fat(ketosis), lose weight and improve overall health status, then this eating plan can give great satisfaction.
- Cholesterol Reduction: LDL better known as bad cholesterol, which deposited in the arteries reduces the proper passage of blood, responsible for the onset of inflammation and numerous diseases (Diabetes, Dementia). The keto diet helps reduce insulin levels and thus the risks of increased LDL.
- Improves cognitive function: recent studies have shown that the keto diet can improve brain function to the benefit of those suffering from neurodegenerative

diseases (Alzheimer's, Dementia) as it stabilizes LDL bad cholesterol, improving blood flow by re-flowing vessels that were clogged.
- ➢ Stabilizes blood sugar: the state of ketosis, stabilizes your blood glucose levels, this means having less swings and fluctuations, you can then avoid experiencing hypoglycemia or hyperglycemia.

Keto...Kick Start

There are many ways to start a keto diet; there is no need to include any particular food or use special varieties of ingredients; you can use foods that you are already familiar with and like.

Be sure to keep track of macros (the total amount of calories derived from carbohydrates, protein, and fat) and calories consumed to stay within the recommended ratio of fat, protein, and carbohydrates.

To help you understand Ketosis, you can find several online calculators designed to help you determine your daily required macro intake, based on your personal data, very useful tools for those starting out.

If you want to try this diet, keep in mind that it can take a few weeks of trial and error before you find the right balance. If you use the recommended keto calculator, you can make a lot of progress without going crazy with calorie counting.

Maximum carbohydrate intake of 40 g/day, recommended for starters, to be adjusted downward once the state of ketosis stabilizes.

Suggested percentages:

10% from carbohydrates | 25% from protein | 65% or more from fat (vegetable).

Tips for Success

It takes patience, from the first day of keto, to obtaining visible results, weeks will pass, changing and adjusting the body's metabolic systems is not a simple task, and it is very individual one. The benefits of the ketosis state are generally felt after 4-12 weeks.

Keep track of macros and calculate the volume of calories to avoid going over or under your daily limit; also, record when you have seizures and check your food intake.

Deviate as little as possible from the basic diet recommended by the keto calculator to get the results you want; as long as you follow the macros and stay within the recommended ratio of fat, protein, and carbohydrates, results will be positive.

Consider alternating your diet: only foods high in fiber, fat or protein for one day and avoid carbohydrates for two days; in this way, you will become more familiar with the foods that satiate you the most.

Weight loss is slower than expected, keto is a different way of eating; therefore, do not expect the same results as an ordinary diet, focus on making a sustainable long-term change, follow your macros, consume enough calories to maintain a steady weight and enjoy food at the same time.

The keto diet is ideal for those who want to regain or conquer body lightness because it helps control emotional hunger, once the body adapts and starts using fat(ketones) instead of glucose, so don't worry about eating, in the keto diet, you eat often and regularly.

Side Effects

Constipation

Constipation is due to your daily fiber consumption being too low. Be sure to consume fiber daily, exercise regularly and hydrate properly as this will promote efficient elimination of waste. If constipation persists, contact your health care provider, and consider taking a fiber supplement.

Bad breath

Your body will begin to release ketones through the exhalation process, which can contribute to bad breath; increasing your intake of foods that promote better oral health, such as parsley and peppermint; using a tongue scraper; frequent brushing of teeth after meals; and daily flossing are all practical and functional solutions.

High uric acid levels

Excess uric acid in the body is linked to cardiovascular disease. Uric acid in the body starts to rise when you consume a lot of carbohydrates, you can reduce this risk by eating more foods rich in fiber, (fruits and vegetables) and low in added sugars.

Irritability

A very common side effect at the beginning of the state of ketosis, which can be traced to a state of dehydration or excessive salt intake, it's important to drink enough water and you can add some fresh lemon juice too, plan to exercise, and as a result achieve extraordinary calming effects.

Achieving Ketosis

The most important step is to make sure you are consuming the right foods needed to stay well and perform all your daily activities without any energy dips.

Balanced consumption of protein is especially recommended, so that you can provide your liver with the measured supply of amino acids for gluconeogenesis. Whether you are following the standard keto diet or the modified Atkins diet (which lasts from 4 to 8 weeks), your goal, primarily, is to achieve the state of ketosis.

To do this, you have to maintain a constant caloric intake, and avoid carbohydrates as much as possible, failing to achieve the state of ketosis, means you are not taking in the correct type of foods, cyclically, and it is possible to experience this difficulty.

When it comes to achieving ketosis, there are essentially two methods. The first is the targeted short-term ketogenic diet that lasts about 5-6 weeks.

The second method is to slowly transition into the diet, gradually decreasing carbohydrate intake over a period of 10-12 weeks, thus allowing the body to slowly adapt and start using ketones instead of glucose as fuel.

Limiting carbohydrate consumption (maximum 20-50 grams/day) helps to decrease the amount of glucose and insulin in the blood, stimulating the liver to release fatty acids that are stored, so they are converted into ketones.

Increasing the intake of good fats (butter, olive oil, coconut oil, avocado oil) promotes and speeds up the human body's entry into the desired ketosis.

Schedule daily physical workouts, increase endurance slowly, stabilize ketosis and help maintain muscle tone..

Ketogenic Foods

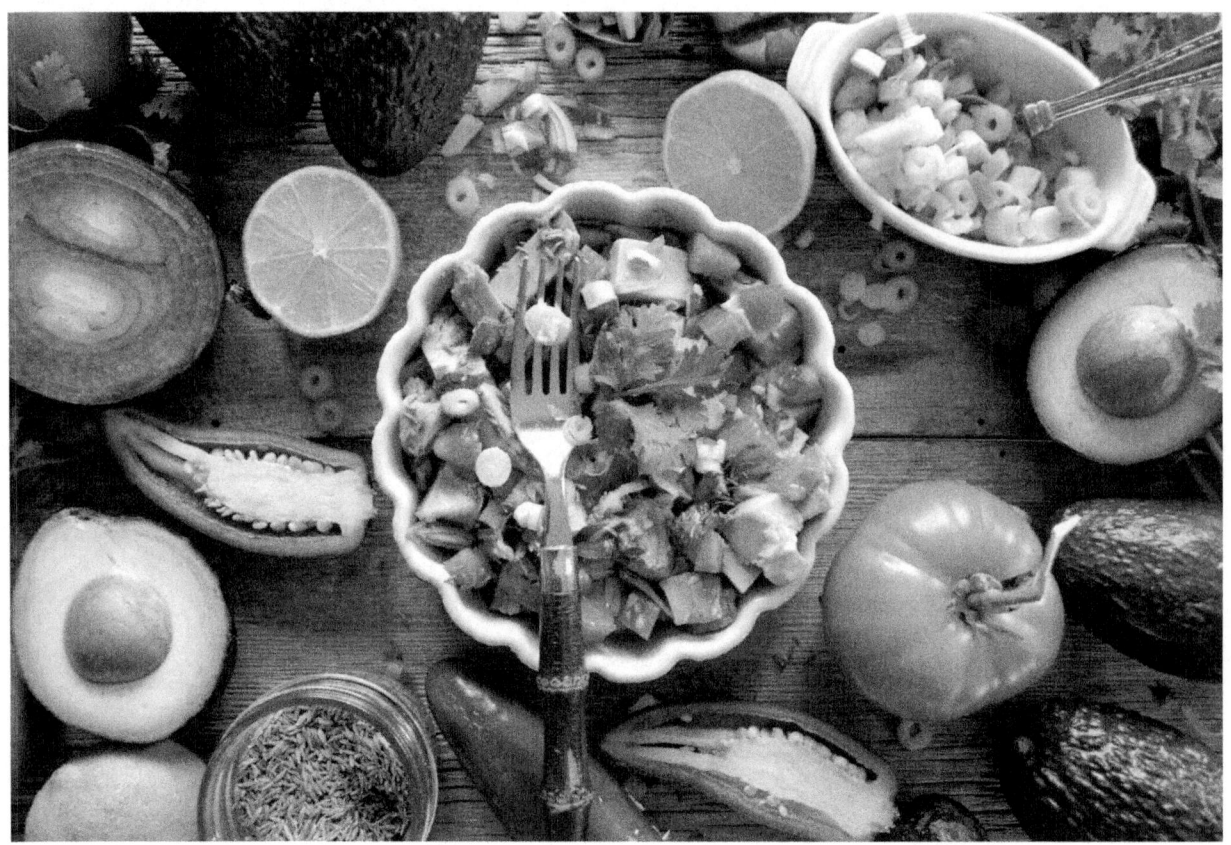

High-fat foods are recommended when starting the keto diet, since fats act as the primary source of energy, instead of glucose.

Tips:

Fats: should account for about 60-70% of total daily intake, recommended nutrients are avocados, butter, olive oil, dairy products, nuts.

Meats: excellent sources of protein and also fat (chicken, pork, lamb, beef) be sure to select fresh meat instead of ready-made packaged products as these contain high levels of salt and chemical preservatives that are to be avoided.

Fish: excellent source of protein and omega-3 fatty acids (mackerel, sardines, cod, sea bream, sea bream, snapper, caught and not farmed fish) Omega-3s are incredibly important because they help the brain and nervous system function at their maximum potential.

Eggs: good source of protein and many other important nutrients, recommended to start the day because they provide plenty of energy over a long period of time. Consume eggs from organic sources if possible, free-range are also a healthier option.

Fresh Vegetables and Fruits: valuable for their fiber content, taken daily, they also act as a laxative. Vegetables and fruits are also a great source of minerals and vitamins, including potassium, calcium, magnesium. The best sources of fish are white cod, mackerel, anchoes', wild tuna, red snapper and salmon.

Eggs: Eggs are an excellent source of protein and contain many other nutrients too. They are a great way to start the day as they provide lots of energy for a long period of time. Look for whole eggs from organic sources where possible as those from chickens raised in warehouses have been shown to have higher levels of cholesterol and hormones that can be harmful to you.

Vegetables: Vegetables contain fiber, which acts as a laxative after eating them. They can be eaten daily or in portions on a weekend. They are also a great source of minerals and vitamins, including potassium, calcium, magnesium, and more.

Healthy Fats

Choose fats that are saturated rather than polyunsaturated ones because trans fats can be bad for your heart. You only need small amounts of saturated fat in your diet as high amounts won't provide you with many benefits.

The best sources of saturated fat are:

The best sources are:

- **Coconut oil:** alternative condiment with incredible health benefits, can be used in different ways to add extra flavor or nutritional value to food, will also help with weight loss, research shows it reduces appetite and increases energy by increasing metabolic rate.
- **Avocado oil:** strategic condiment for skin care, internal organs and overall health, very similar to extra virgin olive oil, if consumed regularly it increases folate (tissue and cell regenerators)
- **EVOO:** extra virgin olive oil, consisting of more than 70 percent monounsaturated fat rich in antioxidants, polyphenols, Omega-6, Omega-3 and fatty acids, which contribute to the perfect functioning of metabolism. It's a favorite ingredient for the liver, which easily uses it to achieve and maintain the state of ketosis.
- **Macadamia nuts:** contain a high percentage of monounsaturated fats, including palmitoleic acid, which promote increased optimal fat metabolism in the keto diet.

Keto...Foods to Avoid

- **Flour, bread, pasta, pizza, etc.**
- **Carbonated and sugary drinks**
- **Potatoes**
- **Industrial and packaged sweets**
- **Added sugars**

Industrial and packaged fruit juices and syrups

The keto diet absorbs the body's fat reserves as fuel for numerous daily activities. It is an effective way to lose weight and improve health, and has many other advantages over the common low-carb diet.

It becomes necessary to eat more healthy fats (saturated fat), take correct amounts of protein from meat, and drastically reduce carbohydrate intake by avoiding all starchy vegetables (potatoes, corn, or other starchy vegetables).

Take in Moderation

- Fresh vegetable juice.
- Berries (blueberries, raspberries, or strawberries) small amounts every day.
- Dark chocolate (70 percent or higher).
- Good wine in small amounts is allowed

Macronutrients for Keto

Keto is the most popular low-carbohydrate diet; in fact, it involves taking about 10 percent of calories from carbohydrates, 25 percent from protein and more than 65 percent from fat.

Macronutrients versus total calories from food:

- **Fat:** 65% or more calories
- **Protein:** 25% or more calories
- **Carbohydrates:** 10% or fewer calories

Fewer carbohydrates and greater amounts of vegetable fats and proteins stimulate the production of ketone bodies in the liver, which are then used as fuel(ketosis) in the muscles and brain.

Keto Rules

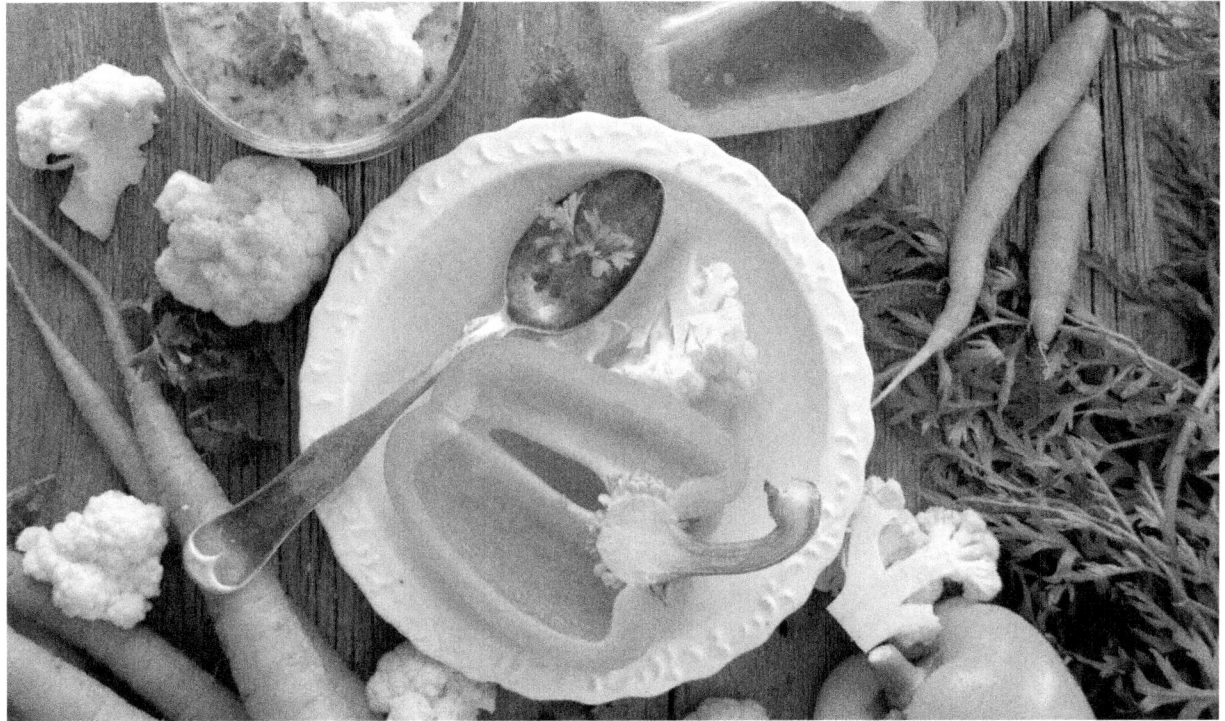

1. Maximum 30-60 grams of carbohydrates per day, protein in any amount you want, nutritious and satiating, especially good for losing weight without constantly feeling the hunger pangs.
2. Avoid starches and stay away from: potatoes, pasta, bread, farinaceous...
3. Make sure to control consumption and vary the source of animal fat (white meat, red meat, sliced meat).
4. No restrictions on vegetable fat intake, so healthy oils (avocado, olive, coconut, flax, chia seeds, nuts, dried fruits).
5. Good wine in moderation.
6. Remember that excess carbohydrates are converted to glucose, which will make it difficult for the body to move into ketosis.

7. Measure your ketone level with a breathalyser or use a glucose meter to monitor your blood sugar.
8. Drink plenty of water, tea, infusions, without sugar to make sure you stay hydrated and avoid constipation.
9. Do physical exercises daily, gradually increasing your endurance to efforts and toning your muscles helps to maintain the state of ketosis and also psycho physical fitness

Meal Tips

Meal prep is recommended when starting the keto diet, rereading the list of foods allowed or to avoid you will find that: vegetable fats, meats, dairy products, vegetables, and fruits are always to be included in daily meals.

It's also very important to prepare high-fat snacks and avoid carbohydrates.

Don't forget vegetable fats...

The important thing is to learn how to eat properly and have the flexibility and variety so you don't get bored. Keto breakfast in the morning will satisfy you for longer and also increase your strength levels and mental clarity.

Follow these basic tips, you won't need much else in terms of ingredients: protein (eggs, fish, meat), vegetables (broccoli, cauliflower, kale, onion), good monounsaturated fats from avocado, coconut, olive or flax oil and cheese, nuts and dried fruits.

How Much Protein Should I Eat?

It is important to get enough protein into keto diet, this can be achieved by eating meat, fish and dairy products in variety, foods such as, sardines and cottage cheese are rich in calcium and perfectly in keto.

The human body uses protein to keep muscles toned, repair muscle and cellular tissue, the amount and quality of exercise planned in the dietary program will determine how much protein your body needs, normally protein intake should be about 1.5-2 grams per kg of body weight.

To be really precise, you will need to calculate how many calories your body requires daily, with the help of the Keto Calculator.

A good rule of thumb is to take in 0.8 grams of protein for every pound of lean mass (body weight/fat), this figure is determined by subtracting your body fat percentage from 100 percent and multiplying by 0.8.

Tips for Managing Leftovers

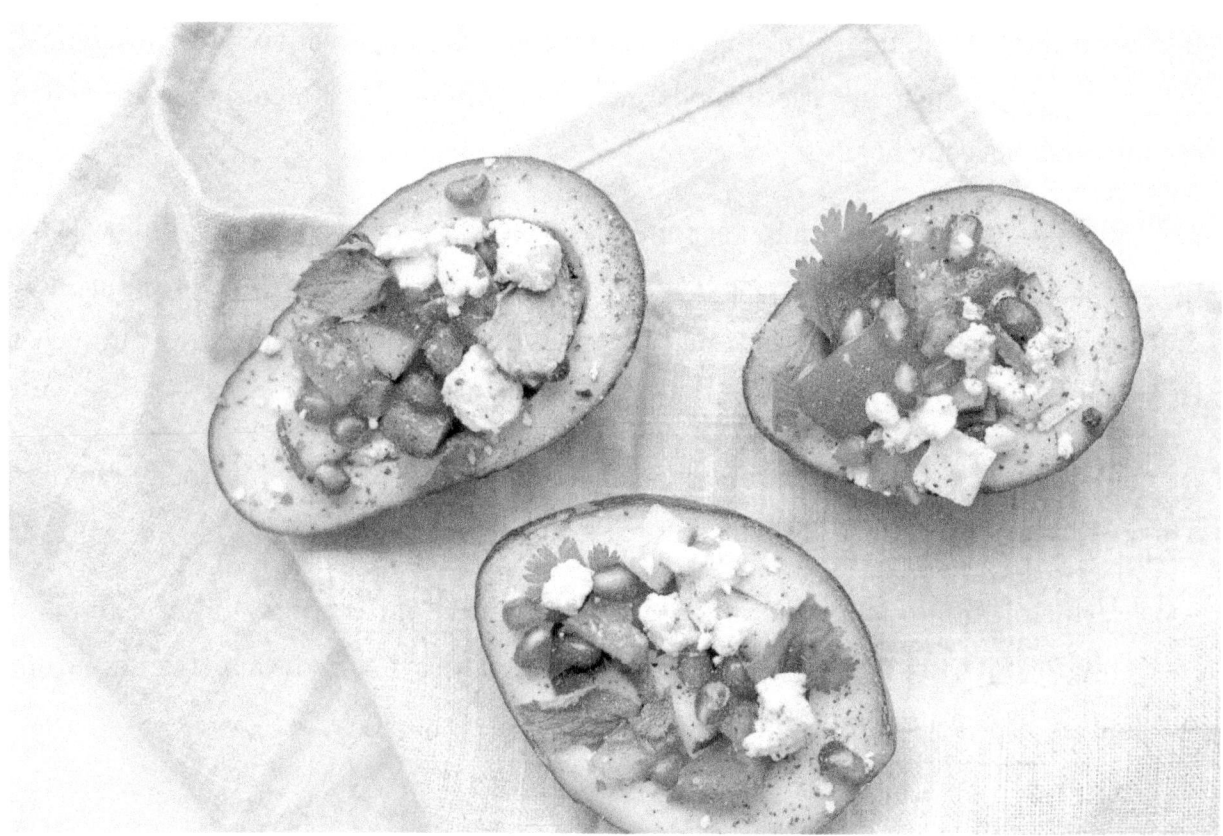

Leftover food is a great resource in cooking or dieting; you can use it to make delicious recipes, soups and salads, meatballs, omelettes, etc.

Here are some ideas for managing leftovers from your meals:

- ➢ They can be used for 3-5 days. If you want to keep them longer, then freeze them in small portions in specific containers.
- ➢ Creativity, you can make a quick and tasty meal out of leftovers.
- ➢ Use them in different recipes such as soups, salads, meatballs, omelettes or preparations to put in the oven.

- By cooking twice, the amount of food you need, you can freeze some of it for another meal, resulting in gaining time that you can use to exercise or just to relax

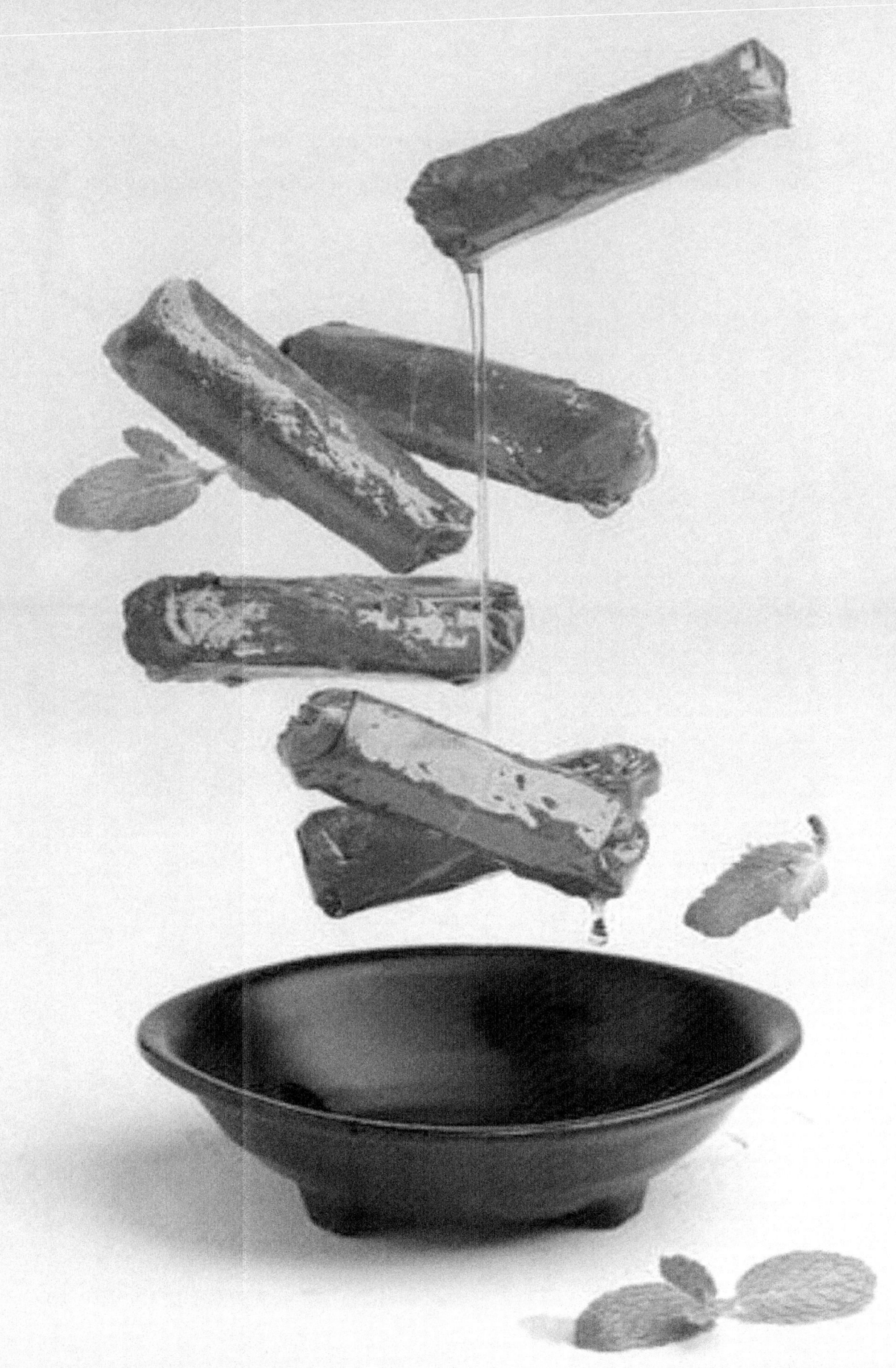

2. Mind and Body at 50+

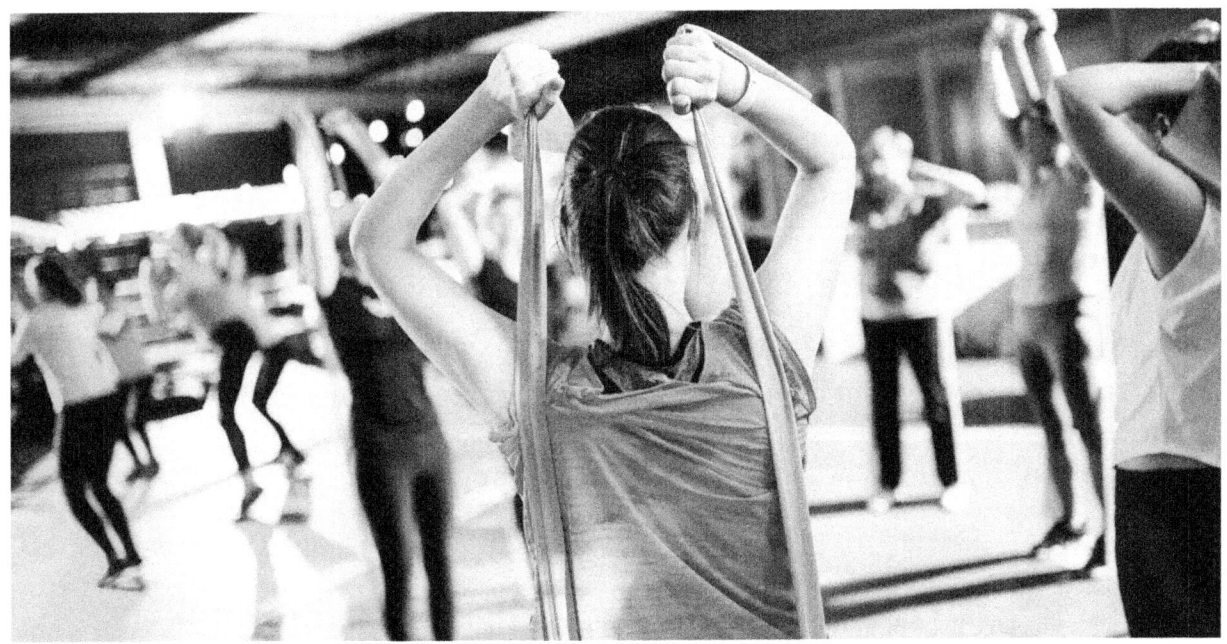

As we get older, several changes occur to the human body, brain, and our judgment of ourselves. Changes that affect our priorities, cognitive abilities, behavior, physical performance, body composition, the way we eat, etc.

Changes in the body at 50+

As we approach and pass "middle age" we need to stay active and maintain good habits, it is vital to eat well, read, and exercise, for example: walking, swimming, bike rides, yoga or free-body mat exercises, etc.

There are many exercises you can do in your 50s, if you attend a gym and use weights as a form of training, then there are methods and machines to lift weights with fulfilment without causing injury.

Focusing on cardio training by doing dedicated exercises such as exercise bike, or relaxation and meditation such as yoga, are some good suggestions to keep your body and mind fit even after 50.

Another way to stay healthy is through diet, eating fresh and unprocessed foods, eggs, fish, meat, vegetables, fresh and dried fruits, balanced nutrition helps keep bones firm, muscles toned and mind active.

Exercise increases appetite, improves mood, decreases anxiety and stress, which increases satisfaction with the meals one consumes; small, frequent, calibrated snacks throughout the day prevent bouts of nervous and emotional hunger.

Common body changes as we approach and pass the age of 50:

Weight gain

When you reach and pass the age of 50, you will experience changes in your body weight, this can be due to several factors that need to be known and verified, among the most common being that you eat more and become more sedentary and your weight increases

It is important to remember that this is natural and should not be a cause for anxiety. If your BMI, (body mass index) a parameter that relates body mass to an individual's height, stays between 19 and 24, it means that diet and training are balanced resulting in an average body mass and relatively good health of the individual.

Formula to calculate BMI: body mass (kg) / height squared

The body mass index of an individual weighing 75 kilograms, with a height of 1 meter 70 centimeters will be:

$$75 / (1{,}70 \times 1{,}70) = 65 / 3{,}4 = 22{,}06$$

Menopause

On average, after the age of 45 in women, a physiological event involving a large decrease in estrogen levels that can cause symptoms such as hot flashes, night sweats, mood swings, and more.

Weak hearing

Caused by the aging process, it is more common in men, depends greatly on the pathologies present in the individual, lifestyle, habits and whether or not subject to vices (smoking, alcohol, eating disorders, etc.)

Taste

The sense of taste naturally tends to decline after age 50, this may be caused by the slow and inexorable reduction of neurons in the brain, but again, it is very much related to environment, pathologies, lifestyle, and habits.

Poorly toned muscles

As we age, it is very common to witness a decline in muscle mass tone. While this is a natural and normal process, it can and should be countered with the right diet and constant physical training (even light exercise)

Obesity

If you are overweight and have a BMI of 30 or higher, it can be a cause for concern, because other health problems may arise; obese individuals tend to have higher risks of inflammation, heart disease, stroke, diabetes, and even some types of cancer.

Skin wrinkles

As the years pass, the skin begins to lose collagen and elasticity begins to decrease, the natural consequences are wrinkles and loss of skin texture. The environment, air pollution, sun exposure, and daily maintenance are key determinants of the lasting health of our skin.

Joint and muscle pain

There are many changes in the human body that can affect the joints. Unhealthy habits, predisposition, sedentariness, old age, of course, cause the joints to begin to weaken, causing pain…often in the knees, ankles, back and femoral area, but also shoulders, neck, and arms, all highly utilized parts of our body. Carrying out daily exercise is always highly recommended…the results can be extraordinary (at all ages)

Osteoporosis

Osteoporosis is a systemic skeletal disease that increases bone fragility and inclination to frequent fractures, caused by resorption of bone mass and deterioration of the microarchitecture present around the bone tissue itself. A typical aging-related disease, it can be countered with, awareness, physical training, balanced diet, healthy habits, and perseverance.

Mind at 50+

Along with the physical-functional changes, cognitive-behavioural changes also begin to appear; it is crucial to understand that this is a normal irreversible process related to aging. The causes are always the same, multiple, as are the solutions, important to act, following the universal action-reaction principle.

Memory loss

Memory begins to be impaired as time progresses, the hippocampus region of the brain naturally begins to shrink and deteriorate as the years go by. Mnemonic exercises, crossword puzzles, healthy sleeping habits, a balanced diet and daily training...are powerful countermeasures.

Sense of smell

As with the sense of taste, which naturally declines with old age, the part of our brain that processes smells lose analysis capacity, also worsened by external factors such as air and industrial pollution.

Dementia

Systemic disease that occurs naturally with the aging process, caused by deterioration of brain cells and lack of blood supply to vessels (called "vascular dementia") most often caused by excess LDL. Typical in the elderly, it can cause severe behavioural changes, the solutions are as always many and encouraging.

Sight

Changes common and often occur in people who already have prior eye disease, or who particularly stress the visual apparatus for work. Many forms: night blindness or the inability to see clearly in low light, as well as difficulty focusing on objects from a distance.

Depression and mental health

It is very common for the elderly to experience depression and other mental health problems, meaning that the level of self-confidence and subsequent self-esteem begin to falter by many different triggers. Increasing sociability is vital as is regaining purpose.

Insomnia

Sleep is a delicate and complicated process, a significant role, is played by melatonin, also known as the sleep hormone, the natural ability of the epiphysis to release melatonin, gradually declines as we age. The triggers are always related to habits: work, food, behavioral, environmental, etc. Melatonin supplementation, after consultation with your family doctor, along with constant exercise can be of great help.

Sleepiness

Daytime sleepiness as a consequence of night-time insomnia. It is common for 60+ people to switch from monophasic to multiphasic sleep, that is, to incorporate an afternoon nap into their daily routine.

This practice can be a solution and at the same time cause serious problems, the main factor is to not confuse sleep with wakefulness, deep sleep is restorative, wakefulness absolutely not.

Importance of training the muscles and mind

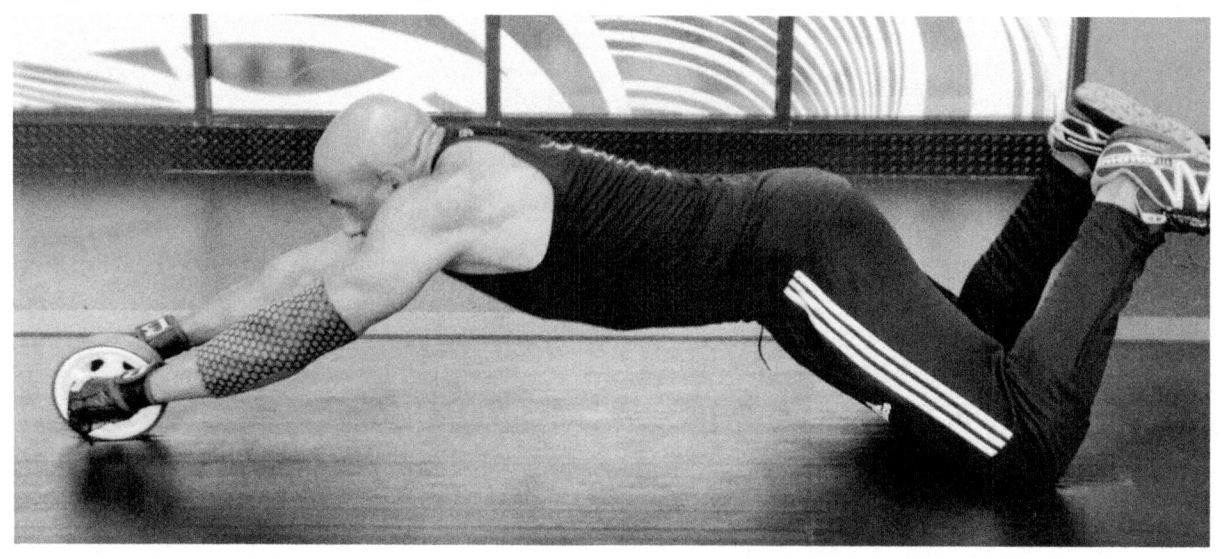

After the age of 40, muscle mass begins its natural decline (Sarcopeny), this means gradually losing physical "strength" as well. Pathologies such as arthritis or fibromyalgia, do not help to find an effective solution.

It is very helpful to incorporate exercise as a daily habit, thus increasing blood circulation and enabling blood to flow to the muscles. The muscles will return to contracting and doing their natural job, restoring greater strength, better balance, and good mood to the affected subjects.

Push-ups

A great way to keep fit while sending blood flowing to the muscles and strengthening them, it is recommended to start slowly with only 5 or 10 push-ups the first time and then increase as you get used to them. Push-ups can be done on the arms and also on the legs (squats) both exercises are great for increasing strength and balance.

Cardio

Cardio is the best way to increase the exertion capacity of the heart and to get the blood flowing throughout the body. At home or gym try an exercise bike or light running on a treadmill, walking outdoors surrounded by nature, bike rides and swimming in the sea or pool are a true medicine for long life.

Speed walking

Perfect exercise for all ages, it is a very effective cardiovascular workout that promotes blood flow and relief to the whole body. Speed enhances the beneficial effects and it is recommended to keep the speed between about 3-5 km/h, for at least 40-60 minutes every day, 2-3 times a week.

Swimming

Swimming is another excellent form of cardio that can be done effortlessly. Swimming correctly and frequently gives great relaxation and benefits to the body and mind. There are many other water-related physical activities, at any city sports center or online you can search and find the workout you like best.

Yoga or free-body exercises

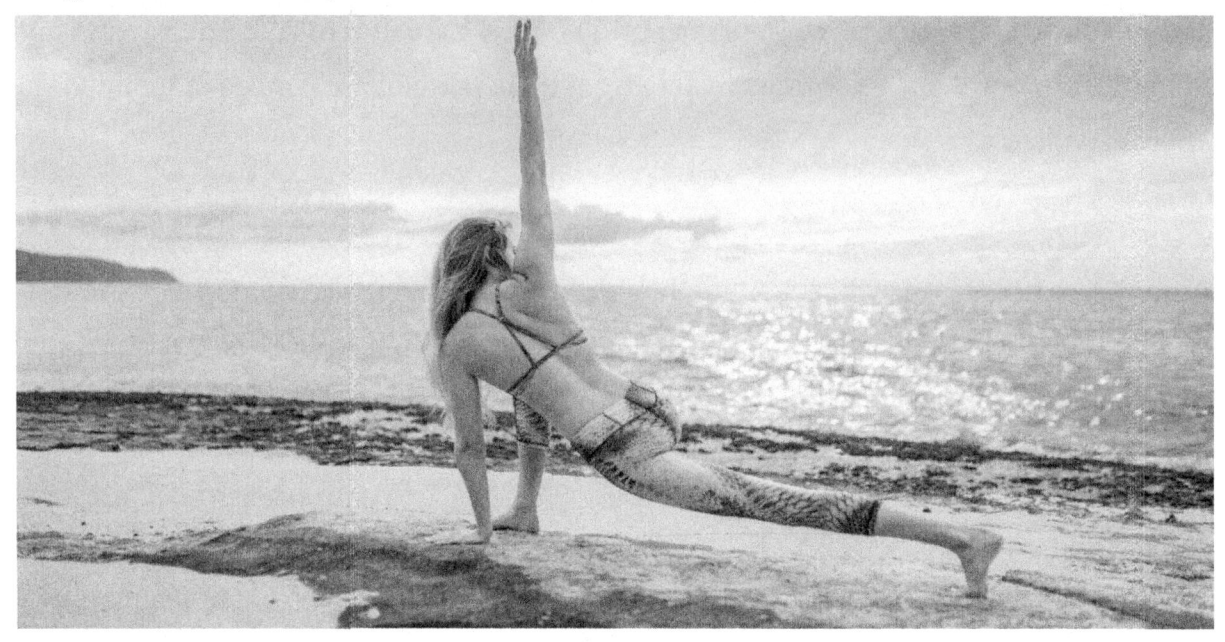

Popular and extremely efficient way to train body and mind at the same time. Helps strengthen many different areas of the body and allows for increased joint flexibility, balance and overall strength. A therapeutic, soothing, and mentally restorative workout for all ages.

Cycling

Feeling the wind and the sun on your cheeks is a priceless feeling of freedom, on a motorcycle as well as a bicycle. Pedaling is environmentally friendly and healthy, offers mood positivity and mental satisfaction, if practiced regularly and with the necessary moderation, tones the muscles.

The lower limbs are more stressed, needing to be kept stronger as they age, thus enabling safe balance in daily movement and newfound confidence.

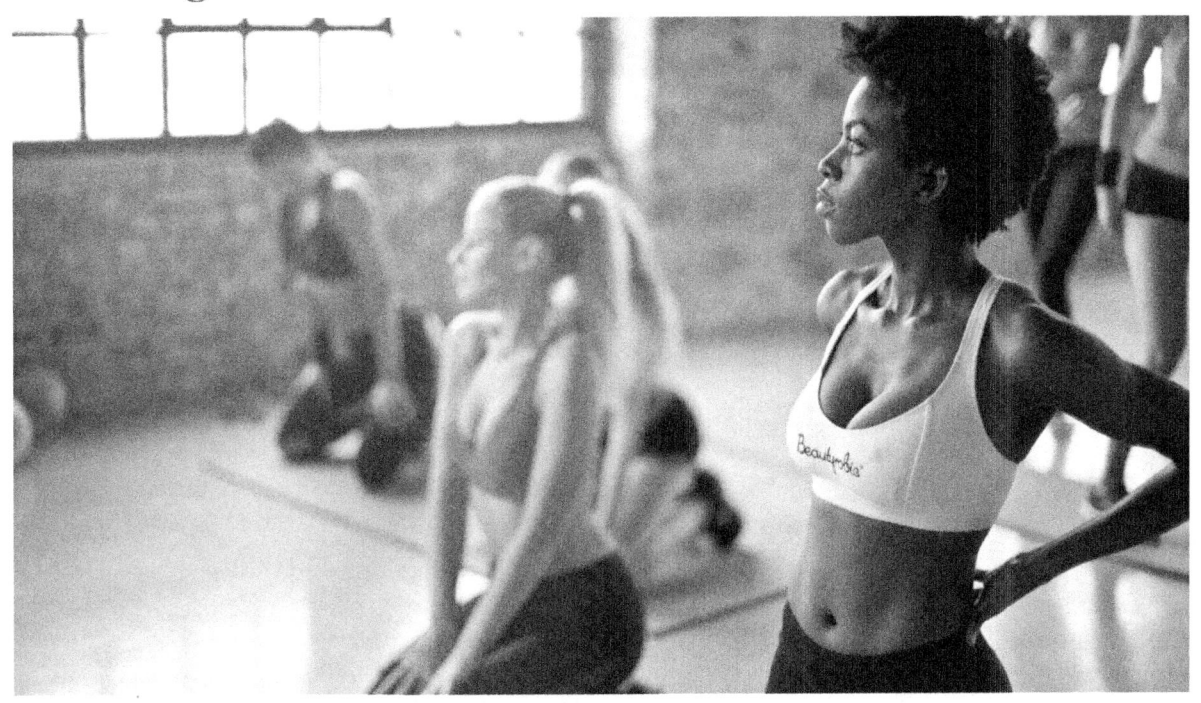

Stretching

Stretching is a de-stressing and soothing way to relieve your muscles after the strain of exercise; it will allow you to relax and stretch your muscles and gain more flexibility in your joints.

Proper diet

The priority is the psychophysical health of the individual, nutrition plays a key role, balanced intake of micro- and macro-nutrients helps to provide the daily energy needed by the body, maintain efficient and functional internal organs, avoid or soothe inflammation, boost immune defences to successfully fight external threats (bacteria, viruses, chronic syndromes, diseases, etc.)

More information and patience, facilitates changes in the diet of adult-mature people. This often happens when they drastically reduce the consumption of pasta and red meat and focus on vegetable fats and proteins.

The reasons for this choice are many and easy to find by inquiring on the web, the massive health benefits, and environmental impact among the most substantial and clear.

Adult people find ways to inform themselves more thoroughly and focus on consuming foods that are as natural, organic, biological, traceable to the source of production as possible. Avoiding harmful chemical preservatives or ingredients that are toxic to health.

This virtuous and shareable behaviour helps prevent the emergence of inflammation, pathologies and numerous other health problems resulting from improper nutrition.

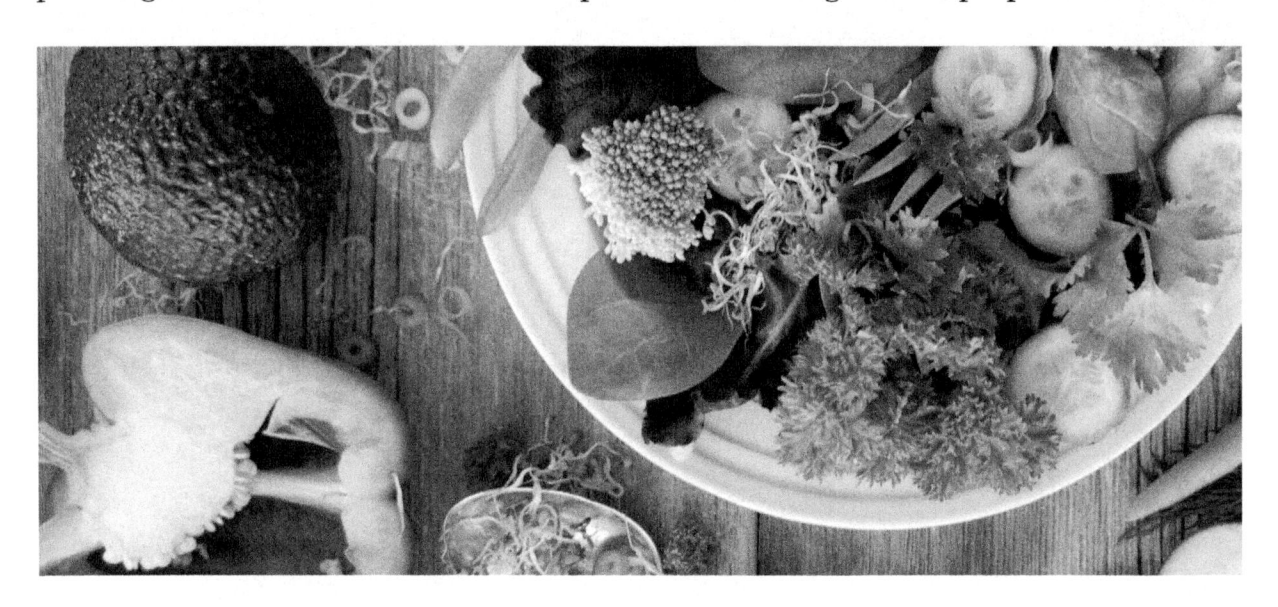

Fast, ready-to-eat and packaged foods

If you want to maintain a healthy body and mind over time you should avoid processed foods which contain chemical preservatives, excesses of salt, sugar and unnatural seasonings.

Remember that every exception confirms its rule, therefore, allow 2-3 days per month for nutritional-emotional transgressions, especially at the beginning of a new diet.

Limit alcohol and sugars

Once you advance in age, it is more difficult to metabolize alcohol, it is therefore necessary to drastically reduce consumption thus avoiding numerous health risks. On the same line, it is important to limit or eliminate added sugars, which are responsible for countless inflammations; excess sugar consumption causes the pancreas to produce less insulin, a protein hormone that is essential for maintaining optimal health.

Eating fruits and vegetables

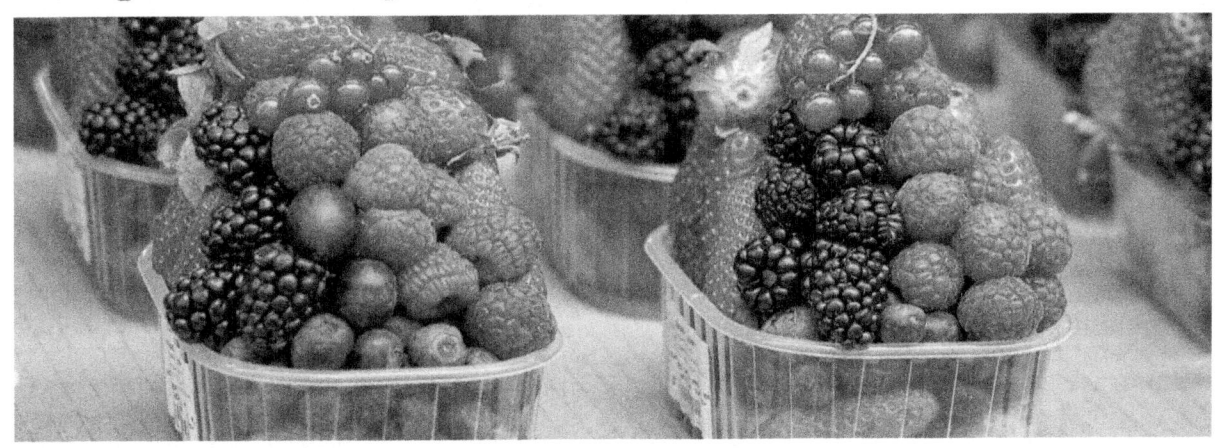

A balanced, daily intake of fresh fruits and vegetables provides the body with nutrients (fiber for digestion and elimination of waste) that are useful for optimal functioning. Dried fruits and raw vegetables are good snacks, optimal for supplementing and feeling full throughout the day.

Dinner 7 p.m.

Are you interested in discovering a method that will allow you to successfully tackle any eating plan?

Ensuring proper nutrition and digestion, involves setting a precise time and menu each day, in order to steer clear of improvisations, thus moving forward quicker along your roadmap. Starting dinner around sunset time, will help stimulate better digestion and promote better and sounder sleep.

Plant and animal fats

Here we come to the keto "mantra," by following this dietary method, the human body gradually learns to produce energy with **chetones** (produced by the liver by synthesizing fats) instead of glucose (sugar extracted from carbohydrates).

Once the individual achieves the desired state of **Ketosis**, the source of energy becomes existing fats (waistline, excess fat legs, arms, etc.) or fat intake, resulting in losing unnecessary weight quickly and feeling better.

Protein is the main player, primarily, in managing the subject's muscle tone and overall strength, so it is indispensable and recommended.

Carbohydrates should not be eliminated completely, because they are vital in the correct human metabolic process, but they should be reduced significantly, as mentioned above.

Water

Drinking an average of 2 liters or more of natural water per day helps to increase satiety', eliminate toxins from the body, and keep the kidneys healthy by eliminating waste products. Checking the sodium, potassium, and magnesium contents in the water you buy and comparing them to charts for the perfect intake of these salts in the body is a good, recommended habit.

Avoid salt and sugar added

Many adults-mature adopt low-sodium diets because, excess sodium causes high blood pressure and leads to endless complications. It is suggested to avoid added seasonings as much as possible, especially if there is disease or inflammation, you should learn to use ingredients, herbs, and spices in your recipes to give flavor, same recommendations with sugar.

Enjoying Food

If you don't like what you are eating, what is the point of eating it?

It doesn't matter if it is cooked impeccably, feeling bored or irritated while feeding yourself is detrimental to your health. The purpose of nutrition is not only to produce energy for the body...it is also plays an emotional role...to enjoy the food and the moment; therefore, be sure to eat what you like and always taste food you are not familiar with.

Keto for 50+

The keto diet is a nutritional method, as we have read, that involves eating very low in carbohydrates, medium in protein, and high in fat.

The Keto diet has an "immune-modulating and anti-inflammatory" effect on the adult-mature human body and turns it into a fat-burning machine; the muscles break down fat to use it as energy instead of glucose (carbohydrates).

The liver converts excess fat, into ketones, which are used as the primary fuel, instead of glucose. This state, called, **ketosis**, is achieved by drastically limiting carbohydrate intake (to about 10 percent of total calories) and replacing it with protein and vegetable fats.

The metabolic state of ketosis helps keep an individual healthy and alleviate-relieve symptoms of various diseases: diabetes, epilepsy, cancer, chronic inflammation, Parkinson's, Alzheimer's, and more.

Professional Tips

Advice from your family doctor or a professional nutritionist will ascertain your health condition before, during, and after the diet and determine the right intake between fats, proteins, and carbohydrates based on your health status and constitution.

Adult-mature people with health problems should seek the advice of professionals who are familiar with the negative or positive effects of diet in relation to existing conditions, so as to avoid choosing a diet that harms rather than promotes the individual's well-being.

Cholesterol

LDL or "bad cholesterol" in the blood is the oxidized low-density lipoprotein, consists of plaque deposits on the walls of arteries, tightening their circumference, obstructing proper blood flow, leading to a condition commonly called atherosclerosis.

Obese adults should try, after consulting a nutritionist, a ketogenic diet, which promotes improvements: it decreases LDL, stabilizes high blood pressure, soothes the effects of diabetes, and helps in losing weight steadily and fast, while dizzyingly decreasing heart strain.

Recent research has related diets and their balance of fats, proteins and carbohydrates, confirming that the drastic decrease in carbohydrates compensated with the excessive intake of animal fats and proteins recorded a significant increase in mortality; in contrast, nutrition with vegetable fats and proteins, records a considerable increase in longevity.

Let's not overlook the prominent role of vegetables in the healthy diet, consuming moderate amounts of vegetables and fruits regularly, ensures the right intake of fiber, which is crucial to avoid and soothe inflammation.

Keto & Aging

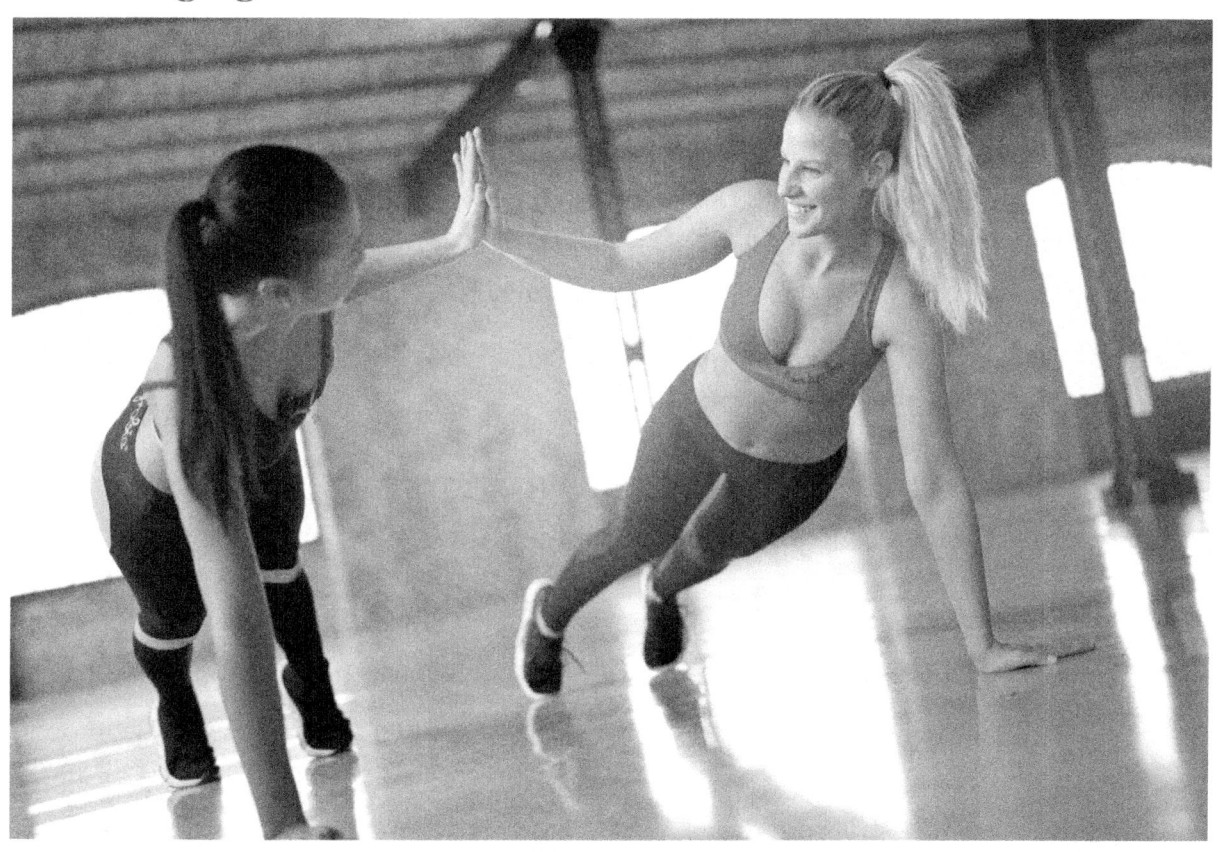

As we get older, we tend to lose physical and even mental flexibility, we become more and more averse to change, often, we lose the lucidity needed to be assertive about the choices we are compelled to make on a daily basis.

Learning new things and being curious are essential to continue living to our own satisfaction and that of the people around us: embarking on a new diet a new healthy habit, eating less, better and more frequently, is the way to start off along a new path on the right foot.

You'll experience less fatigue, less pain, more satisfaction, more physical lightness and mental clarity thanks to the increased energy levels due to ketosis. In just a few weeks or months, you will notice a substantial difference both physically and mentally.

Ketosis Effects

The human body switches to using fat(ketones) as fuel rather than the carbohydrates(glucose)that your liver and muscles used before. This process dramatically decreases weight and provides more energy to carry out daily activities, while also improving mood and strength.

The state of ketosis tends to improve blood pressure, decrease LDL levels, decrease states of inflammation, anxiety and stress, and promoting physical activities.

Studies on the keto diet show relief in disorders such as panic attacks, bipolar depression, epilepsy, migraines, and chronic pain. Keto has the potential to reduce inflammation and alleviate many neurodegenerative diseases such as Alzheimer's and Dementia.

Keto & Hormones

Hormones are chemical messengers; they originate in the endocrine glands, carried by the blood, they activate actions within the body that stimulate biological reactions.

For example, as we grow and age, the decrease in estrogen levels leads women to menopause; testosterone levels, in men, usually decline gradually.

Reduction of growth hormone leads to shrinkage of muscle mass with loss of strength. Low melatonin implies loss of normal sleep-wake cycles (circadian rhythms).

The keto diet acts, essentially, by regulating 2 key energy-managing hormones produced by the pancreas are: insulin and glucagon. keto has been shown to be remarkably effective in regulating insulin and stabilizing blood glucose.

Recent studies conducted on women diagnosed with PCOS (polycystic ovary syndrome) who regularly follow a ketogenic diet show a significant improvement in reproductive hormone and insulin levels, increasing fertility in those struggling to conceive.

It is important to work with your family doctor or a professional nutritionist, who, knowing your health status, are able to advise you on the best dietary course according to your somatotype, constitution.

Keto Procedure 50+

Achieving the state of Ketosis, less traumatically and in the shortest possible time will allow' the individual to enjoy and benefit from the positive effects of burning fat reserves and losing weight.

- The rules for entering ketosis are simple:
- Drastically reduce carbohydrates
- Regularly feed on fats and proteins several times a day
- Give preference to plant-based fats and proteins
- Take in fresh seasonal fruits and vegetables regularly
- Exercise regularly
- Check by testing for ketosis status
- Keep in contact with a trusted nutritionist
- Correct things that are not working
- Consistency and perseverance towards your end goal
- Maintaining and acquiring new healthy habits

Keto Confidence

It is always worth remembering that the keto diet originated as a treatment for childhood and adult epilepsy when drugs were absent or ineffective. Only later, given the very positive results in terms of decreased-appearance of seizures, was it introduced as a low-carbohydrate diet.

keto is not just a dietary method to lose weight, but a lifestyle to soothe, relieve and try to resolve inflammation and chronic ailments.

Be sure to get enough calcium, magnesium, and vitamins D and B12; these nutrients are sources of energy, increase bone strength, positively regulate mood states, and contribute to good metabolic functioning.

New healthy habits at 50+

As we age, our minds no longer work as optimally and quickly as they used to, we forget more things than usual, it's part of the aging process: anxiety, stress, habits, nutrition, existing diseases, etc...

Will the brain continue to lose neurons every year?

What habits should be changed to stem this natural decline?

How can I be sure it works?

No sureness without proof (evidence)

There is no single, painless, effective solution for all people; everyone has his or her own negative habits that he or she struggles to eliminate due to laziness or lack of knowledge.

Negative habits lead to health problems, inflammation, chronic syndromes, diseases and general mental and physical malaise.

Implementing healthy and positive changes in a lucid and conscious manner is a prescient and wise way to face the years ahead.

If not at 50+...then when?

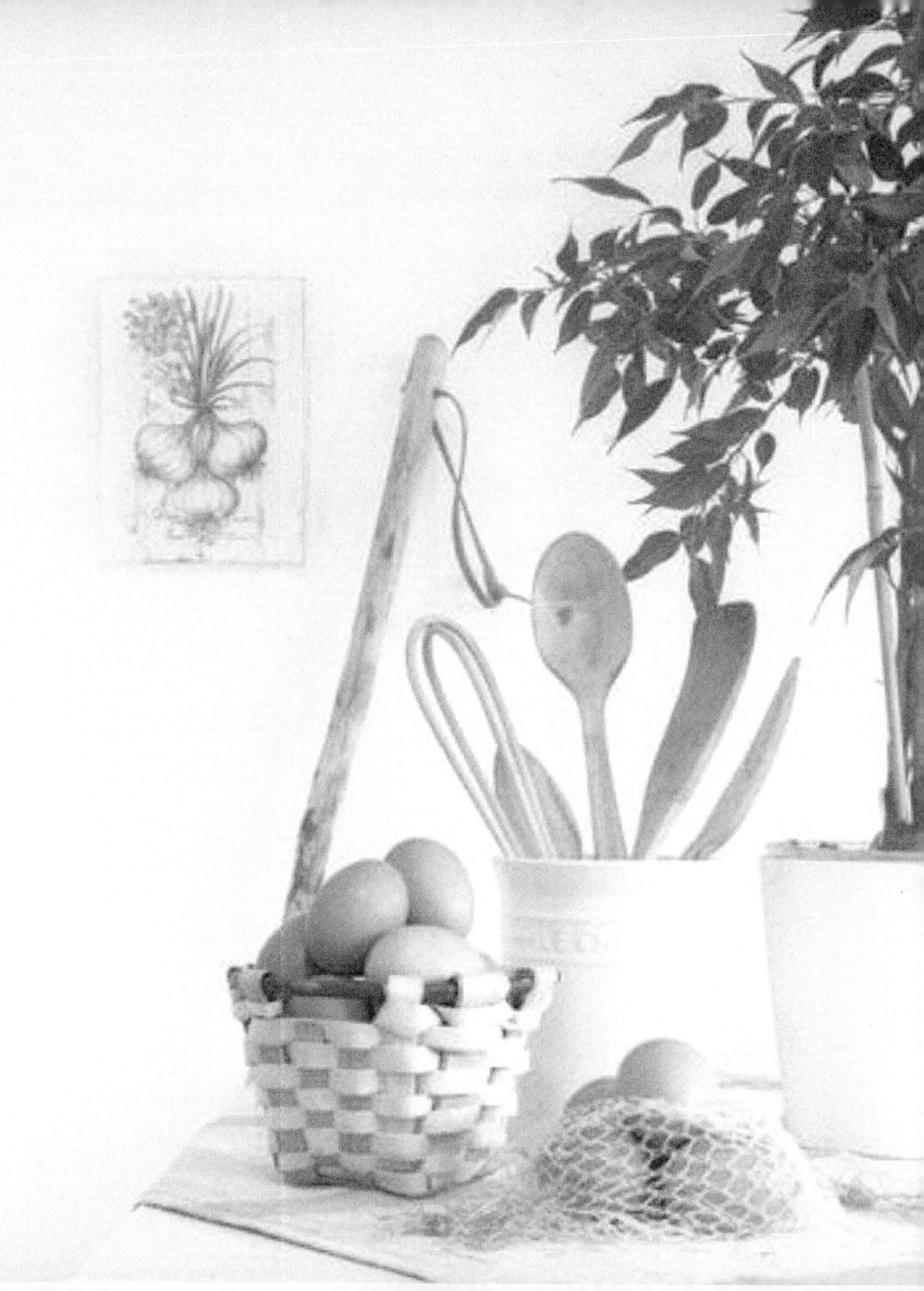

3. Equipment and Tools

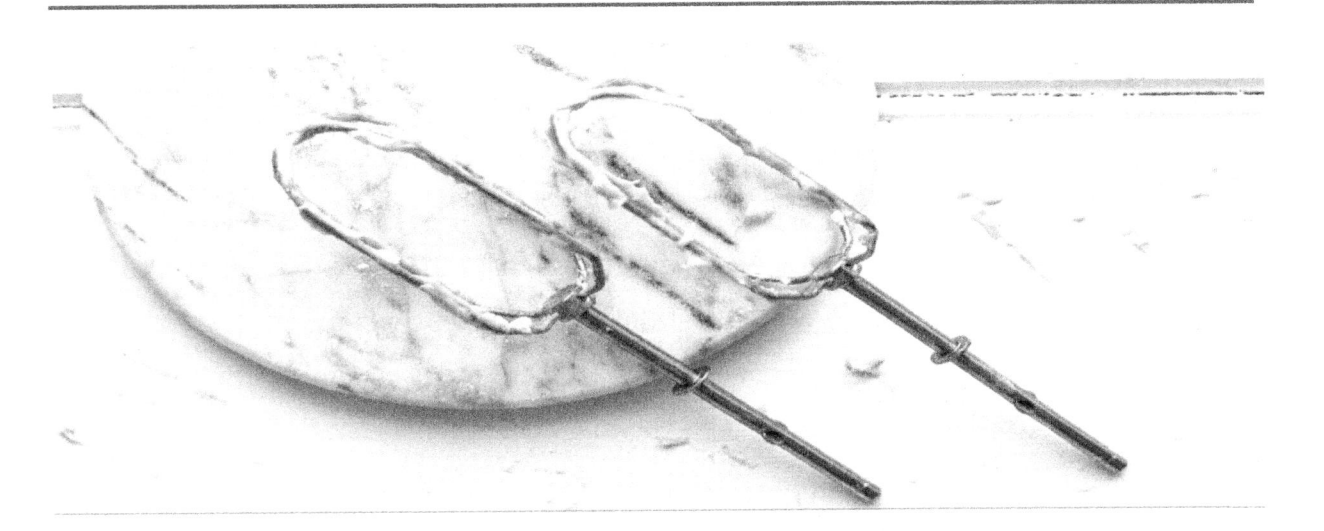

We're going to cover kitchen equipment and gold tips for the ketogenic diet. As a reminder, a ketogenic diet is low in carbs and high in fat content. It's an excellent way to eat if you're looking to lose weight or lower your cholesterol. This is also one of the best diets if you have type 2 diabetes. By cutting carbs from your daily food intake, your body will be sent into ketosis, which burns fat as its primary source of fuel instead of glucose (sugar).

Kitchen Equipment

Here is some kitchen equipment that will help you prepare meals for your keto diet:

1. **Mug:** The best coffee mug for a ketogenic diet is stainless steel. It will keep your coffee warm for hours and help you prepare your healthy meals faster.
2. **Chop-top:** This is the pot that's used to prepare food on the stovetop. The edging helps to keep the contents inside the pot in place, so you don't waste any water, juice, or spices while cooking.

3. **Liquid measuring cup:** If you are buying a liquid measuring cup, choose a glass one over a plastic one as plastic one tends to break easily and may end up leaking your liquid ingredients inside.
4. **Blender:** The best blender for the ketogenic diet is Vitamix. It can grind almost everything you throw at it, including nuts, seeds, and even coffee beans!
5. **Cutting board:** The best cutting board is bamboo or wood. Avoid using plastic ones if possible because it has been found that they are hard to sanitize and may contain toxic chemicals like BPA and Phthalates which are harmful to your health.
6. **Saucepan:** Choose a saucepan with a capacity of 3–4 quarts, the bigger the better as it will save you time when cooking for the whole family.
7. **Mixer:** The one you choose will depend on the food you wish to mix. If you are preparing salad dressing or whisking eggs, go for a traditional hand mixer or immersion blender because they can do the job without the fuss of a regular mixer.
8. **Grater:** The bag grater is great if you are looking for a quick way to get some shredded veggies or cheese into your salad dressings. But if you're using it in the kitchen, safety is of utmost concern, so make sure it's conical, has stainless steel blades, and that it's dishwasher safe.
9. **Cutting knife:** A good quality knife is essential for any kitchen, especially if you're making many salads and green vegetables. You'll need to use it to chop all your ingredients.
10. **Whisk:** Egg whiskers are usually made for mixing the egg yolk and incorporate air into the eggs when making, e.g., Hollandaise sauce or meringue. But they can also be used to mix ingredients in a blender or food processor, like flour, if you are about to make pancakes or bread!
11. **Vegetable peeler:** The best vegetable peeler is one that has a sharp blade and doesn't take off too much of the vegetable as you are peeling it. It's perfect to have

one that removes thin strips that you can use to wrap around the meat to make a nice-looking appetizer.

12. **Meat pounder:** If you're preparing meat for some dishes, it's good to have a meat pounder in your kitchen as it will save you time and energy rather than using your fist or any other utensils around.
13. **Milk frothier:** This is perfect for making a hot or cold mocha latte with your favorite coffee. It can also be used in making thin milkshakes such as a sugar-free strawberry milkshake recipe.
14. **Pastry brush:** This flat brush is ideal for brushing egg whitewash or olive oil onto a dish or pan to give it that lovely shiny finish it requires before cooking.
15. **Cake tester:** If you're baking some cakes, pies, or muffins, it's a must-have kitchen tool that will ensure you have that perfect consistency of the batter and baked product.
16. **Grater with a pouring bag:** This is ideal for grating, pressing, or crushing your zest or citrus fruits into your favorite recipes.
17. **Kitchen scale:** A kitchen scale is an indispensable tool in any kitchen. It allows you to keep track of the amount of food you put in the fridge and helps you with portion control. For instance, if you buy 3 kg of avocados for your next recipe, measure them all out before entering the fridge so that when it's time for that recipe again, you will know exactly how many avocados are left to use!
18. **Corkscrew:** If you like drinking wine, this is the one kitchen utensil that will not only save you a lot of time but also make it easy for you to open those pesky wine bottles.
19. **Julienne peeler:** This is like a regular vegetable peeler, but instead of thin strips, it produces small thin sticks that are perfect for making your own stir fry or salad.

20. **Potato ricer:** If you come across the term "mashed potatoes" on the ketogenic diet, then this is what you'll need! It's a tool for pressing the moisture out of potatoes so they become nice and fluffy.
21. **Scale, salter, or refrigerator:** If you plan to measure or weigh food in the portioned containers, you will need a scale and if it's not digital, then make sure it has a reasonable LCD display with an easy-to-use knob.
22. **Cookie sheets:** The best cookie sheet is one that has easily removable non-stick coating, so your cookies don't stick to it while they are in the oven or once you put them on your plate.
23. **Spatula:** A silicone spatula is ideal for spreading and scraping. It's a good addition to have one of these because you can use it on the stovetop too, rather than just on the baking dish when you are cooking.
24. **Flat measuring cups:** If you like to bake cookies or bread, it's important to measure your ingredients accurately and measure them in the right portions to keep track of how full each container is. It's also important to have accurate measurements so that you don't end up using too much of an ingredient, thus affecting the flavor of your product!

Recommended Foods

When getting started with your keto diet, I suggest you consume the following foods:

- **Healthy fats:** Focus on adding in as much fat as possible and eliminate processed and saturated fat. It's not essential that you consume a lot of animal products as a keto dieter. You can start with consuming some eggs and salmon to get your omega 3s easily from food.

- **Fiber sources:** Add fiber to your diet by eating plenty of green veggies like broccoli, kale, and spinach. These foods act as a great source of fiber and will help to keep your body full.
- **Carbohydrates:** Add starch to your diet by eating vegetables such as cauliflower, zucchini, and asparagus.
- **Fat sources:** You can consume the following forms of fat on the ketogenic diet:
  - Avocados are a great way to get healthy fats easily. They are also super tasty when eaten alone or with some salt and lemon juice.
  - Olives can be consumed in small amounts, but they should not be eaten too often because of the high amount of salt they contain.
  - Olive oil is high in fat as well and it's a healthier option than butter.
- **Coconut oil:** Most people have heard of coconut oil by now because of the various health benefits it portrays. You can use coconut oil as a butter substitute, a massage/facial moisturizer, or a hair glossier! There are many other ways you
- can use it so be creative and start experimenting!

Gold Tips for Ketogenic Diet

- **Eating out should be avoided:** This is something I feel very adamant about because when you're eating out, you are not in control of what you're ingesting. Some restaurants like to add unhealthy saturated fats and sugars into their dishes. If you have no choice, then do your research online and try to find the restaurant that has the lowest amount of fat and sugar in their meals.
- **Carry snacks:** When traveling or visiting someone who is not keto-friendly, it's good to have some snacks in your bag so that you can still stick to your diet with ease.

- **Drink plenty of water:** This is very important and something that's often forgotten. The ketogenic diet tends to dehydrate you. Make sure you drink at least 2 liters a day and add lots of ice to your drinks, so you get more water into your system.
- **Eat whole foods:** When possible, choose whole foods over processed foods. Whole foods contain less sugar and fat, so they are better for the ketogenic diet.
- **Empty out your kitchen:** If you have tons of unhealthy junk food in your home, it will be very easy to simply grab some snacks or meals when you're hungry and it will probably be easier to give up on the diet this way. Try to keep your kitchen clear of excess food so that it's easier to stick to the diet.
- **Do not go back on the diet:** I know that this is something you want, but don't give in just yet. The last time we lost weight, it was easy to start the diet and we didn't have as many cravings when we were eating healthy. However, after a certain point, our bodies started adapting and it became harder for us to stay on our diet. If you've been keto before then I suggest waiting until you reach your goal or pre-set weight goal before going back on the diet. Reduce your calories slightly and start with a low-carb day to see how you feel. If you don't like it, then you are free to go back on the diet.
- **Keep a food journal:** This is especially true if you're not very familiar with what foods contain what nutrients. It's important to keep track of your portion sizes and the calories that you consume each day so that you don't end up eating more than your daily calorie limit.
- **Include physical activity in your routine:** This is important because being on a diet and not moving much can cause you to gain weight. Your body needs exercise so it can burn up fat and keep your metabolism going strong.

Lifestyle Changes with Keto Diet

These are things that I changed in my lifestyle with regards to the ketogenic diet and how I started to feel healthier.

- **I started drinking 8 glasses of water a day:** Drinking water is so important because it helps you to hydrate your body and keeps your body running as smoothly as possible. Many people forget about this aspect of their diet, but the results are astounding, it's easier to stay active without feeling hungry all the time.
- **I started doing yoga:** Many people do yoga at home, but I suggest that you join a local class. Not only will it help you stay active, but you'll also learn some great poses that can be incorporated into pranayama exercises, which are essential for staying healthy on the ketogenic diet.
- **I started sleeping more:** This is so important because sleep will help to lower your cravings. People tend to eat things when they're feeling tired or lazy. Make sure you get a good night's rest because this will help to keep your binge-craving in check.
- **I started taking cold shower:** This is revitalizing for body and brain, releases endorphins, and you have an absolutely great feeling to face your daily routine more energized and focused.
- **I started taking hot baths:** Hot baths are great for burning off excess water in your body and keeping yourself warm during the colder months. They also help to relax muscles and help to relieve pain from soreness or injuries. Baths can be very therapeutic so make sure you try to schedule one every week.
- **I started using yoga-meditation:** I found that meditation helps me feel more relaxed during my day, just start with 10 minutes of long breath and relaxing in butterfly yoga pose (standard pose sitting with your hands clasped on feet,

straight back, heels close to pelvis, bring outer knees down, soles together edge of feet on the floor). It's great for your body and mind so make sure you give it a try!

- **I started keeping to myself**: This might be hard because family is important but if you don't want them to know that you're on a diet (which they shouldn't know in the first place) then just keep them out of it. Your body is not theirs and they should not have any say in what you eat or lose.
- **I started drinking my coffee black:** This is something big that many people do not realize. All the caffeine that you consume goes directly to your liver so when you drink black coffee, you are not taking in so much of the harmful effects of caffeine. You still get your fix of energy and focus from a cup of coffee, but all those unwanted calories are burned off with the caffeine.
- **I started eating more vegetables**: I know that this might sound absurd because everyone loves meat, but certain vegetables have very little fat or calories and can be very filling without feeling full. I still make sure to include plenty of meat in my meals, but I take an extra serving of vegetables and mix it into my meals. I also make sure to keep an eye out for the fat and calorie counts on my items so that I can buy the most nutritious ones to help me stay on track.
- **I started taking multivitamins:** I like selecting vitamins that are good for my body and easy for me to fit into my daily routine. My favorite multivitamin is one from Thorne Research, where they have everything, you could ever want in a vitamin supplement at a great price with no additives or fillers.
- **I started exercising more:** I know that this might not be something you expect to have on your "lifestyle changes" list, but exercising is very important. I suggest that you try to get outside and walk or run every day. Even if it's only five minutes of your day, make sure that you get yourself moving because exercise is the best way to keep your body shape and burn fat.

- **Don't be afraid to get extra help:** If you need extra help with your diet, don't be afraid to seek advice from friends or experts in the field. If you can't get started on a certain diet for whatever reason, then give another one a try. So many diets change over time so you never know what the best one for you will be.

Ketosis is an amazing way to lose weight and improve your overall health, but it will not work for everyone. I like the keto diet because it has been very successful for me, however, it's important that you do your research and understand things such as whether your body can adapt to a high-fat diet. That's why I suggest trying out different ketogenic diets before settling on one that looks appealing to you.

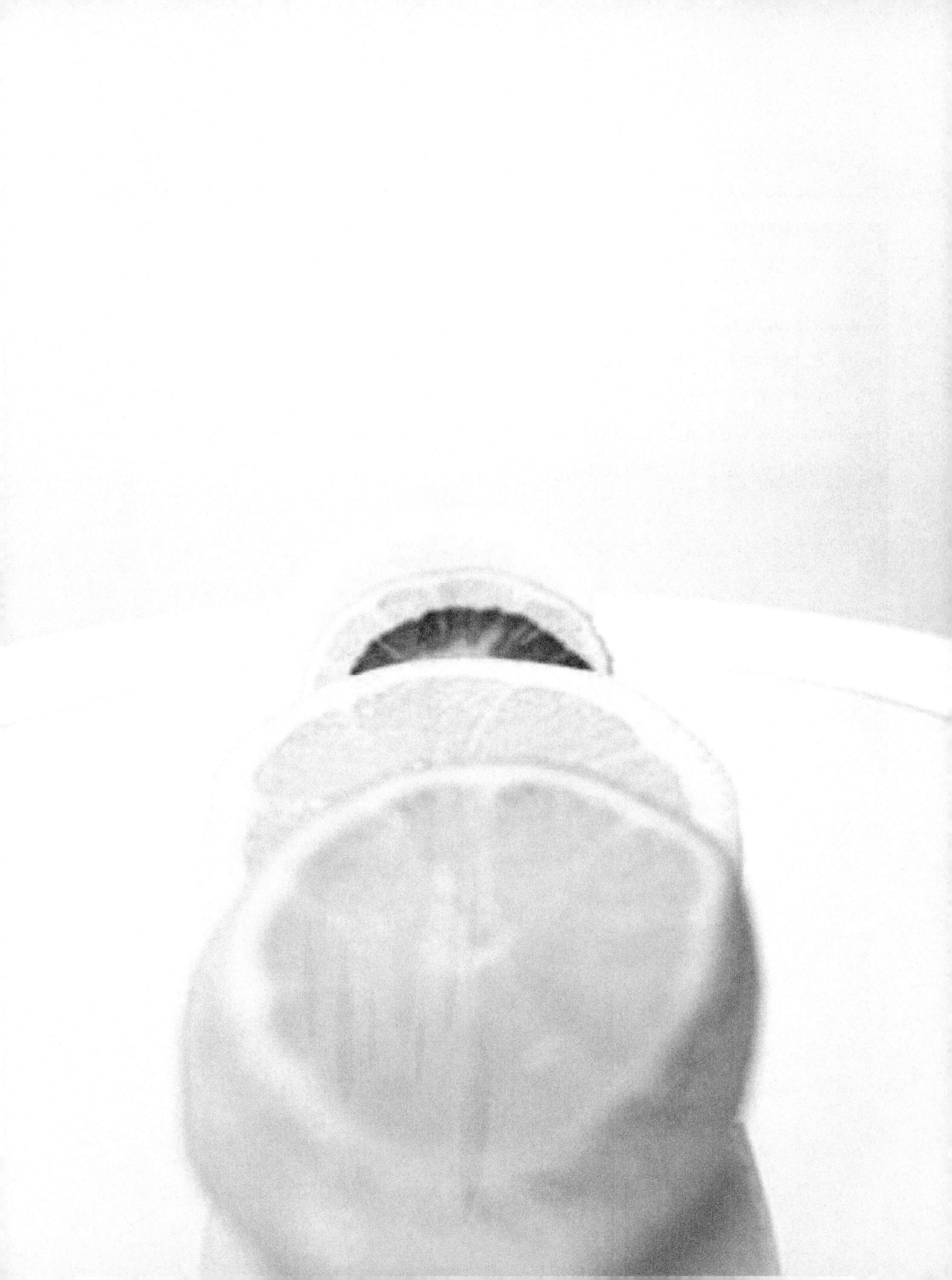

4. Ketogenic Meets Mediterranean

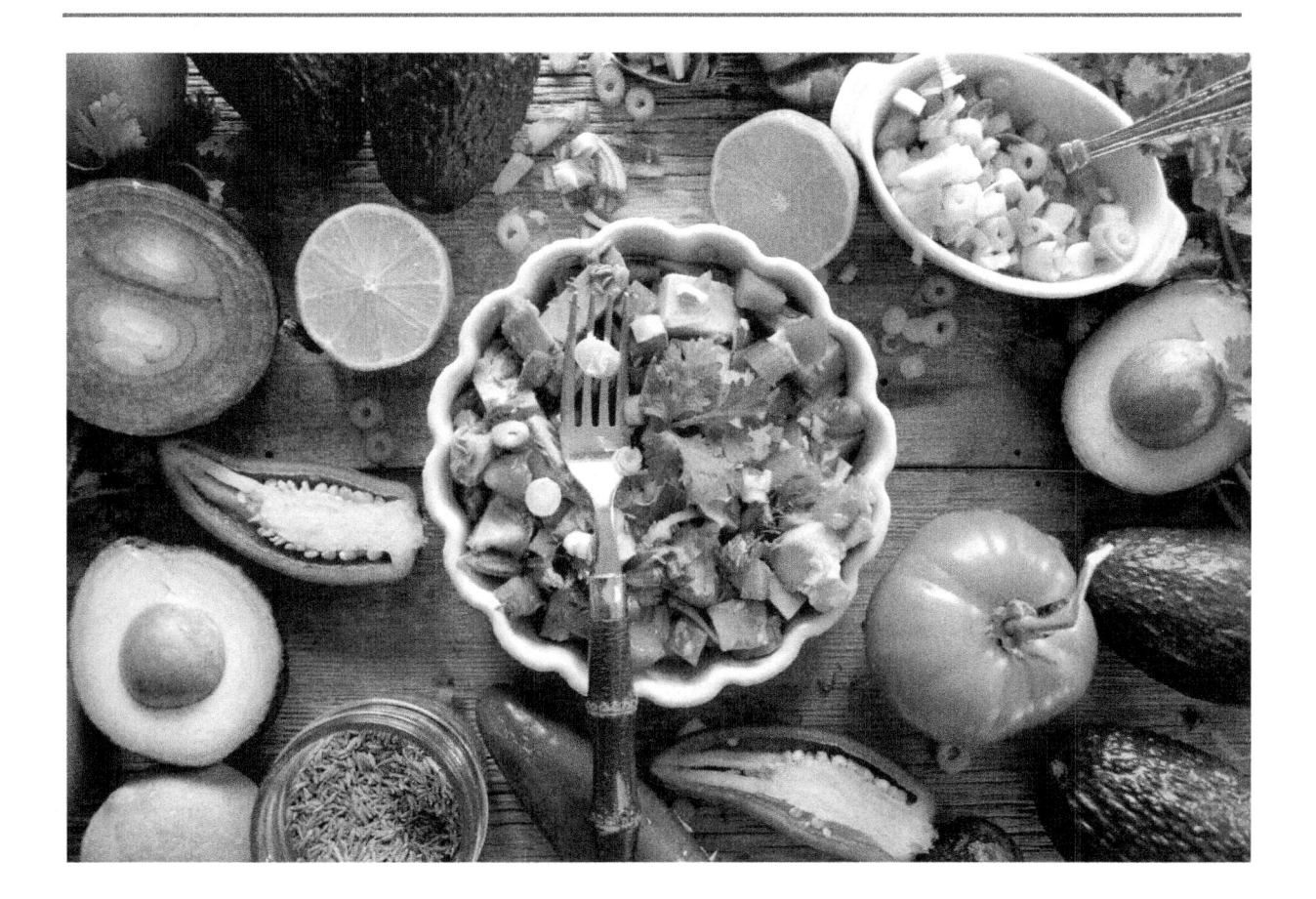

What Is Mediterranean Diet?

Mediterranean-DM Diet

DM is a very specific style of living and eating originating in countries bordering the Mediterranean Sea, it is very popular all over the world because it works, it is widely proven by the testimonies of longevity and health of people who have been using it successfully for so many years. It is protected by UNESCO and in 2010 it was included in the list of oral and intangible heritages of humanity.

Following this dietary method helps you feel better, includes of course, daily physical exercises to keep the body and mind responsive, the use of superfoods is recommended, such as oily fish (sardines, cod, mackerel), extra virgin olive oil, seeds, nuts, caught fish, fresh vegetables, dried fruits, and a glass of fine wine daily.

DM can help reduce risk factors for many diseases, inflammation, cardiovascular disease, neurodegenerative syndromes, about 80% of people who follow this lifestyle and nutrition (widely confirmed and known statistical data) live longer and better than people who do not follow or do not know this method.

One of the secrets of DM's success is consuming foods low in saturated fat, avoiding convenience or packaged foods, industrial baked goods, snacks, fried foods, carbonated drinks or soda, and excess animal protein.

Does DM promote weight loss?

There is no clear-cut, black or white, answer to this question-it is a matter of priorities and what an individual wants to achieve from an eating plan, if it is only weight loss (more than 4 kg per week) then the Mediterranean diet is probably not the right diet, eliminating fat accumulated from years of bad habits, involves time and hard work.

The high fiber intake and low-calorie nature of this diet do not make it suitable for rapid weight loss; it may be the case that overconsumption of animal fats and proteins, bread, pasta, pizza, farinaceous foods, EVOO condiments, and sugars leads these people to gain weight.

Balancing, and scrupulous attention to food plans will promote the achievement of the much-desired weight loss, in the time it takes, to maintain the strenuous results achieved with the help of daily physical training.

DM, scientific research shows, is linked to decreased risks of cardiovascular disease, general inflammation, chronic syndromes, neurodegenerative diseases (Parkinson's, Alzheimer's, Dementia) when used as a nutrition and lifestyle for a long period.

However, it is always wise to evaluate these results with emotional detachment because it is unclear how much of these benefits are direct consequences of DM and how much is due to other factors, such as physical activity, healthy living habits, environmental pollution, attitude to change, and perseverance.

DM & Keto Analogies

In terms of general nutrition, DM shares many similarities with Keto. Both diets are high in healthy fats, vegetables and fiber, animal and plant proteins, excludes added sugars and salt, and avoids convenience, packaged and industrial foods.

However, it is correct to note that the Keto diet is not always compatible with a Mediterranean method-the very low carbohydrate intake and lack of grains are contrary to the principles of the Mediterranean diet.

As opposed to the Keto diet, DM is not restrictive in food choices and does not require calorie tracking or other similar tasks.

Fish is the suggested protein source in DM, which is undoubtedly also a recommendation in the Keto diet, eggs and white meats and cheeses are present in both diets, even selected red meat can be consumed in different proportions in both diet plans.

DM emphasizes the consumption of plant proteins (beans, lentils) which does not align with Keto; however, a Keto-Mediterranean diet can be achieved by keeping carbohydrate intake around 50gr per day.

Keto and Med may have both health benefits, but they differ in their approach to micro- and macronutrients. Selecting which eating style to adopt, a person should consider his or her priorities: weight loss, psycho-physical health, and pathology prevention, that said, several issues of DM can be applied to the Keto diet with encouraging results.

DM & Keto differences

The Keto diet is generally used by people who want to lose weight fairly quickly and still enjoy a wide range of allowed ingredients. DM has a long track-record, proven by scientific data, to have the ability to improve psycho-physical health, as a result of weight loss and increased longevity and quality of life of individuals.

DM is very flexible, does not require monitoring of calories and is not that restrictive with daily macronutrient ratios. It allows a balanced daily consumption of carbohydrates, healthy fats, and fine wine, while also recommending frequent physical activity.

The Keto diet, on the other hand, is very restrictive with carbohydrates and changes the metabolism fuel from glucose to fat(ketones). It requires a challenging adaptation to the physiological state of ketosis, going through a weakening of the individual by Keto Flu (Chapter 1)

The differences are mainly in the results in the medium to long term. Whereas the Med diet has a proven history of success and maintenance, in contrast to this, keto works, proven by scientific evidence, in the short to medium term, as a therapy against obesity, but we do not yet have data and experience on the long term.

DM & keto compatibility

Keto diet originated as a medical therapy, the protocol of VLCKD, the set of all Keto, suggests the use for a short period of time, implying a dietary reworking of the subject achieving metabolic flexibility, after this phase, DM could be adopted as a method of nutrition for the long term.

It is possible to cross the Keto and Med diets, focusing on the consumption of green leafy vegetables, healthy fats such as EVOO and Avocado and Walnuts, a balanced intake of animal protein (fish, meat, cheese) while also considering a share of carbohydrates (50gr-day) and fresh fruits (blueberries, raspberries, blackberries, etc.)

The main feature of Keto is to reset the metabolism, the individual is induced into a physiological state (ketosis), which allows fats(ketones)instead of sugars(glucose) to be synthesized as an energy source for the whole body.

The Keto-Med diet, combined, has several benefits and these increase over time, as the body adapts to the new physiological state(ketosis), Keto-Med attacks fat mass, protects lean mass(muscle), and greatly reduces the feeling of hunger. One can see a dramatic decrease, particularly noticeable in the troublesome abdominal fatty areas and blood circulation and blood sugar also improve.

The Keto-Med diet plan sums up the benefits of both diets and eliminates the differences, helping to achieve relatively fast weight loss with maintenance of psycho-physical health in the medium to long term.

Keto-Med Diet

Let's make an obvious assumption: it makes no sense to set the two diets against each other to reduce a health-related topic, to a form of competition just makes one want to smile...which is also good for you.

Instead, we can grasp the beneficial rules from both diets and put them into practice, likewise avoiding the penalising rules, all with the aim of achieving psycho-physical well-being of the individual approaching this specific dietary method.

The Keto-Med diet is an improved combination of the 2 diets, with a higher ratio of healthy fats, in terms of specific health benefits. It's also less drastic and is more acceptable to individuals sensitive to their body's transformation from a carbohydrate(glucose) burner to a fat(ketone) burner.

This eating plan is more sustainable long term, it is not determining "how much you eat, but what you eat". After the shock of weight loss, our body and mind need to be guided on a path of adaptation and settling into the new eating plan and new body weight.

Keto-Med is a nutritional method that can give optimal results for the individual's lifetime.

Keto-Med Directions

The Keto-Med diet is characterized by 3 phases.

1 **Restoration**: comparable to restoring the functions of our PC or Smart Phone when problems occur, we need to do the same thing with our metabolism as well...but, a few minutes or half a day's work is not enough.

We need at least 4 weeks to cleanse the liver (dandelion infusions and herbal teas) and start the diet: reduced carbohydrates (30gr-day), proteins(70-90gr-day) fats(90-100gr-day) light daily physical activity, morning meditation to fight anxiety and stress.

We enter the state of Ketosis and learn how to manage the new method of energy production calmly and patiently, lose weight (5-6kg) using fats, it is the most important stage for the success of the whole journey.

2 **Adaptation**: after struggling to achieve the first goals, a 4-week stabilization phase is needed again, where we reintroduce a higher percentage of carbohydrates (60gr-day) fresh fruit (blueberries, raspberries, blackberries) gradually from the third week we introduce legumes (beans, lentils) and whole grains (Oats, Spelt, Rice).

At this stage it is very important to continue daily exercise, walking briskly, cycling, swimming, yoga, free-body exercises and meditation, the body and mind will adapt better to the new diet, and you will feel more vigorous and peaceful.

3 **Maintenance**: i.e., monitoring and maintaining the well-being achieved, metabolic flexibility regained, then, our metabolism can again run on the 2 main fuels (Glucose and Ketones) depending on the presence of one or the other in our body...great right?

It is at this point that we can adopt the Mediterranean style, making sure to always consume a higher percentage of fats than carbohydrates, to facilitate the state of ketosis, without anxiety though, because now we know how to quickly switch from one fuel to the other (ketones-glucose and vice versa)

Let's not forget to hydrate properly, drinking plenty of water is a secret to the lasting success of our psycho-physical well-being, water with the right amount of mineral salts with fixed residue around 500 mg-liter, and to continue regular daily exercise, mind you.

Keto-Med Benefits.

- more energy and less hunger than other low-carb diet plans.
- significant decrease in body fat, thanks to ketosis

- blood sugar under control, reduced risk of heart disease, inflammation and diabetes, keto-Med is better for cardiovascular health helps maintain average LDL levels.
- mental clarity, newfound ability to set goals and achieve them, rejoicing in a day out on the bike with family and-or friends, planning a healthy keto Med-style picnic.
- anti-aging effect, using ketone bodies our central nervous system accentuates energy efficiency, affecting the delay of the natural aging process of cells.
- positive mood and moderate optimism are the results of proper nutritional method combined with a healthy way of life, exercise, reading, meditation and acquiring new habits.

5. Nutrition, Workout & Rest at 50+

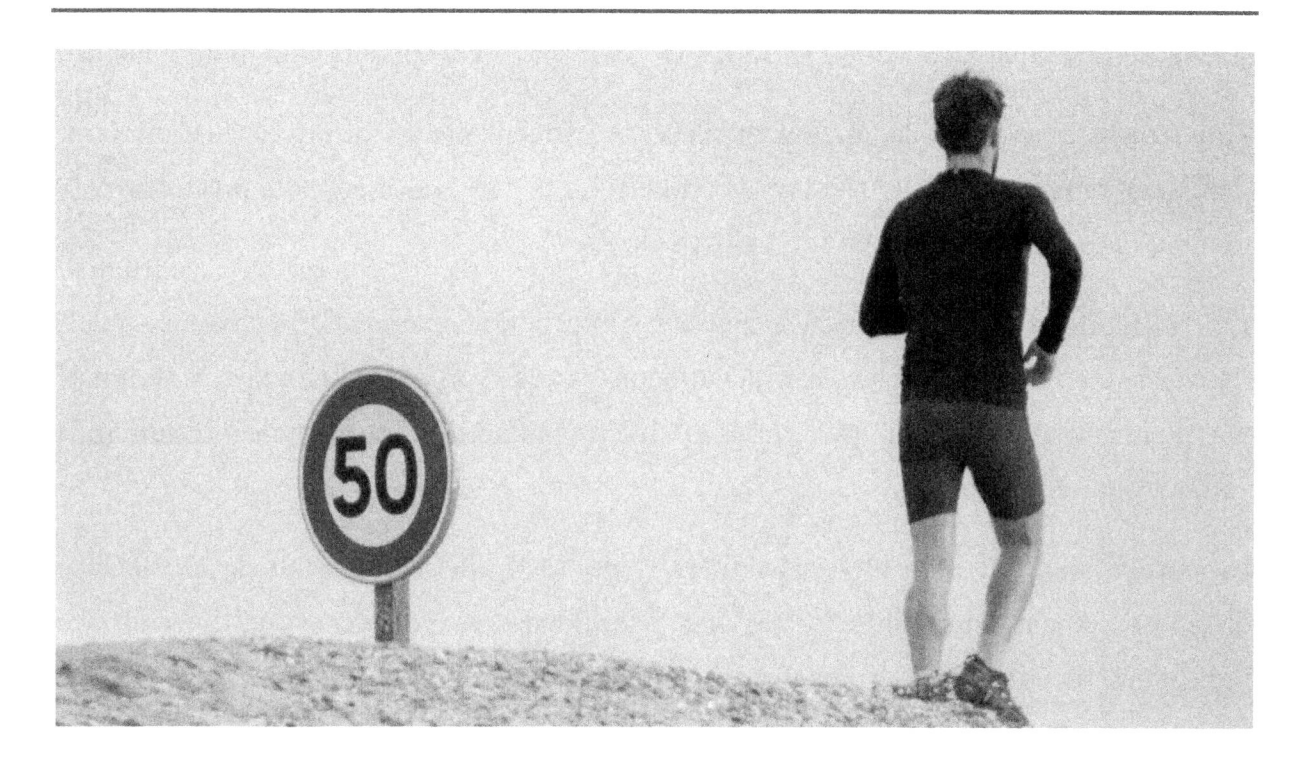

Holistic Approach

Balanced nutrition and good rest-recovery are necessary to train efficiently at any age. At the same time, regular exercise increases motivation, and consequently leads to being more careful with food, and promotes recovery and rest. And again and again, the sequence repeats itself...as 'hunger comes by eating' 'results bring results'.

Get the elephants out of the room now....

The Keto eating plan suggests and allows for low and moderate intensity physical training, while it requires an adaptation period of a few weeks before you can introduce high intensity exercises.

Exercise is a mainstay of mind and body health, during any diet, at all ages. It plays a crucial role in promoting cardiovascular health, maintaining muscle mass, strengthening bones and has an extraordinarily positive consequence on mental health.

Thus, the balanced keto diet makes the necessary fuel available for physical exertion, of low and moderate intensity right away and after a few weeks of adjustment to the new method of nutrition, even high intensity workouts.

Low- or moderate-intensity physical activity, while dieting, increases blood ketone levels and decreases and glucose levels, this happens because you are using body fat stores as energy for physical exertion, and the available fat is mutated into ketones, resulting in losing weight fairly quickly.

In contrast, high-intensity physical activity, temporarily decreases ketone levels in favor of glucose (sugar) and will normally increase blood sugar; the cause is that you are increasing the demand for ready-to-use energy to your metabolism, very quickly, therefore, you will begin to burn more glucose.

By regaining the metabolic flexibility, we had in childhood, we will be able to naturally administer a change of fuel as needed.

By habituating the mitochondria to break down fats to produce energy, with the keto diet, we will burn the sugar we need, getting it from protein, vegetable and minimal carbohydrate intake.

The human body uses the sugar it needs, when it needs it, without reverting to glucose (carbohydrate)-based metabolism, allowing you to:

- ➤ train without suffering metabolic imbalances
- ➤ significantly increase fat synthesis as an energy fuel
- ➤ not affect lean mass(muscle) for energy production.

Physical Activity 50+

Outdoor walking or using a treadmill, outdoor cycling or indoor exercise bike, swimming in the sea or pool, yoga and free-body exercises on a mat are all permitted and recommended activities to achieve maximum results whilst on the keto diet.

Cycling, swimming, and brisk walking are aerobic activities that require an efficient cardiovascular system, and an optimal energy supply that comes from having macronutrients present and balanced in our metabolism.

The keto diet in the first 4 weeks can improve the performance of adult-mature exercisers engaged in these aerobic activities by allowing optimal utilization of macronutrient intakes, increasing resistance to fatigue.

This method of nutrition optimizes body composition (decreased fat mass used as energy) allowing low and medium intensity efforts to be sustained for longer periods of time, with appreciable maintenance of glycogen stores, essential when training intensity increases.

Flexibility workouts help lengthen muscles, better support joints and increase muscle performance, yoga and free-body exercises increase balance and elasticity, preventing injury and relieving the muscle during and after exercises.

Stability and balance exercises, improve alignment, give more strength to muscles, increasing the quality and safety of movements.

An aerobic exercise involves short, intense bursts of energy, such as weightlifting, movements to music, or high-intensity exercises; carbohydrates are the indicated fuel for anaerobic exercise; therefore, the original keto diet does not provide sufficient fuel for these workouts, recommended instead is the Keto-Med diet.

Keto exercises

Which type of activity and at which intensity?

It depends on the somatotype (indicates the constitution of an individual, considering the skeletal and muscular system based on anthropometric characteristics) of each individual, his or her mental and physical health status, and the phase of the diet he or she is in.

Recovery Phase

This phase is useful for resetting the metabolism and preparing, cleansing the liver for the start of the new dietary method. Short muscle toning routines (30 minutes a day 4 times a week) are suggested.

Walk fast, take the stairs, walk as much as possible instead of using the car, find clever excuses to take advantage of physical movement, get off the bus before your destination, take the grandchildren to the park, schedule an aerobic class at the gym or online from home etc.

Increased exercise will be helpful to boost metabolism so that it begins to burn fat, induced by ketosis, and stimulate good balance and equilibrium.

Intense aerobic activity is not recommended at this time because of the scarcity of calories available.

Adaptation Phase

The adaptation phase is characterized by the reintroduction of carbohydrates with a relative increase in available energy; the individual at this point should combine the Keto diet with a more intense aerobic workout.

Suggested is a bicycle or exercise bike ride of at least 60-90 minutes at a regular pace without peak exertion, other aerobic sports (yoga, floor exercises) 2-4 times a week according to a plan agreed upon with a nutritionist and professional trainer.

Maintenance Phase

Maintenance is a phase with many critical issues and should be approached by following the rules scrupulously to avoid making the sacrifices made so far in vain. Increasing calories and energy, it is generally recommended to sustain physical activity every day, alternating aerobic activity, with exercises for flexibility and stability for at least 40-60 minutes each day.

Physical activity and movement are always recommended and encouraged as part of an acquired lifestyle, which allows the individual to reprogram, stabilize and maintain healthy habits, without risking regression...the dreaded and hated yo-yo effect.

Positive effects of physical activity

Lighter, leaner and faster due to the absence of glucose and water (glycogen), which are no longer stored in the body using fat.

A virtuous cycle of using fats and cholesterol, as energy sources, is activated, which increases testosterone levels allowing even more stored lipids to be burned

Fat stores are virtually unlimited, as opposed to glycogen, which means energy in great abundance.

Consume fats (avocados, hemp hearts) before your physical workout so you have an available and quick source of fuel for your muscles.

Also consume protein (Macadamia nuts, Chia seeds, Pumpkin) after your workout.

Supplement with carbohydrates, to balance, in the form of green leafy vegetables that have the virtue of being low in starch and sugar (broccoli, cabbage)

Side effects of training

Do you know your... Why?

And are you powerful enough to motivate yourself in difficult times?

Especially the beginning of a new diet path as keto compromises athletic performance and energy levels, especially in the first few weeks, the body is not yet accustomed to using ketones as fuel, instead of glucose, and that is why you need to be animated with patience, perseverance, and determination.

Muscle mass can be maintained by following a keto diet and more complicated to increase it due to calorie deficiency, this possibility will be postponed when protein and carbohydrate intake are increased.

Finally, it's worth mentioning that the original keto diet is not the most suitable for the purpose of power training and muscle gain, with rare exceptions. The lack of information is still great and the current studies very poor to confirm the continuation of the physiological state of ketosis in the long term.

Recover

The muscle rebuilding phase is crucial and occurs mainly during the recovery rounds from physical activity; muscle recovery means a full day of rest, allowing the muscles to recharge their energy and rebuild. Relaxation, therapeutic massage and deep sleep.

You may happen to suffer from a sleep disorder called Insomnia, which is often caused by anxiety, depression, substance abuse, improper eating habits, absent or insufficient physical activity, and stressful pace of life.

Physical pathological conditions, mental disorders, hormonal dysfunction, drug abuse and intoxication, and unfavourable environmental conditions are countless triggers that require consultation with a professional and thorough expert.

In this chapter we will deal with incorrect diet, hectic lifestyle, caffeine, tobacco, alcohol and other stimulants, which can significantly disturb and disrupt sleep.

Often are the small lifestyle changes that are simply and trivially therapeutic, for example…introducing daily personalized exercise, linked to a well-balanced diet plan custom built on the individual.

Nutrients and Rest

Deep sleep is a sweet and distant memory for the 50+…it's laid back a bit, eh?

Serotonin is the 'neurotransmitter' directly related to good mood, nutrition, serenity and rest, to produce and increase serotonin in our metabolism naturally, is enough regular physical activity, sunshine and light.

Comfort foods, rich in **tryptophan** and sugar, like chocolate, are lead players in increasing serotonin levels that:

- ➢ Increases the feeling of satiety
- ➢ Decreases hunger pangs and thus the amount of food intake
- ➢ Promotes the consumption of protein at the expense of carbohydrates

During the night, **serotonin** is converted by our metabolism into **melatonin**, this 'sleep-defining' hormone regulates the human body's circadian rhythm and is a key player in the synchronization of the sleep-wake rhythm.

Irregular and disturbed sleep reduces ability to concentrate, increases irritability, weakens the immune system and increases the risk of depression and anxiety.

Melatonin plays a key role in regulating and promoting good restorative sleep; this hormone is present in foods of animal and plant origin and can be supplemented by the intake of foods containing tryptophan, zinc and magnesium, vitamin B1 and B6.

Melatonin-rich nutrients:

Oats	Onion	Corn	White Meat
Almonds	Asparagus	Brow Rice	
Walnuts	Legumes	Fish	

And all foods found in the Keto diet.

Keto and Intermittent Fasting (I.F.)

Fasting and Nutrition

The human body is in a state of **nutrition** when we are ingesting food, and in intervals between meals. When we are not eating, the body is in a state of **fasting**.

Decreasing the amount of food consumed, concentrating on eating at certain times during the day, reducing the caloric intake, accustoming our bodies to being without nutrients for unusual and prolonged intervals of time and stimulating and producing positive effects on our bodies, are the methods and benefits of I.F.

The human body begins to use accumulated fat (abdomen, hips, backside) to produce daily energy, as we now know during ketosis, effectively mimicking a state of fasting, given the little glucose in the blood.

During I.F. instead of burning ingested fat, the human body burns stored fat to produce energy for its daily needs.

Keto diet added to I.F. naturally promotes a number of positive reactions on the health of mind and body: during the physiological state of ketosis, the brain works lucidly, thanks to ketone bodies produced by synthesizing fats from our liver.

The abundance of fats ingested during Keto, replaces glycogen with ketone bodies as a source of energy for the brain that boosts and continues its work, it is very common to read testimonies of people (including myself) who feel much more mentally lucid and determined to achieve goals.

The physical training routine leads to a number of benefits too, during I.F., exercising at low and moderate activity on an empty stomach increases athletic performance, maintains muscle flexibility, and promotes rapid absorption of nutrients when eating meals.

Keto + I.F. are ideal for reducing weight significantly, stimulating Ketosis, activating Autophagy (physiological process of cell cleansing caused by I.F.) regaining metabolic flexibility, and naturally boosting immune defences.

The professional nutritionist and the athletic trainer are two empowered partners in our drive to a healthy and satisfying life. We shouldn't hesitate to consult them, listen to their suggestions before starting, and create a relationship of trust and respect, because' our body reacts differently to any treatment (somatotype).

The general rules of Keto and I.F. are the direction to follow, but during the journey, it is normal to experience crises and the onset of doubts about the efficacy, when this happens, breathe deeply and call your nutritionist who will guide you on how get back on the right path.

breakfast
snacks
lunch
dinner
veggies
dips
sweets
fruits

breakfast & snacks

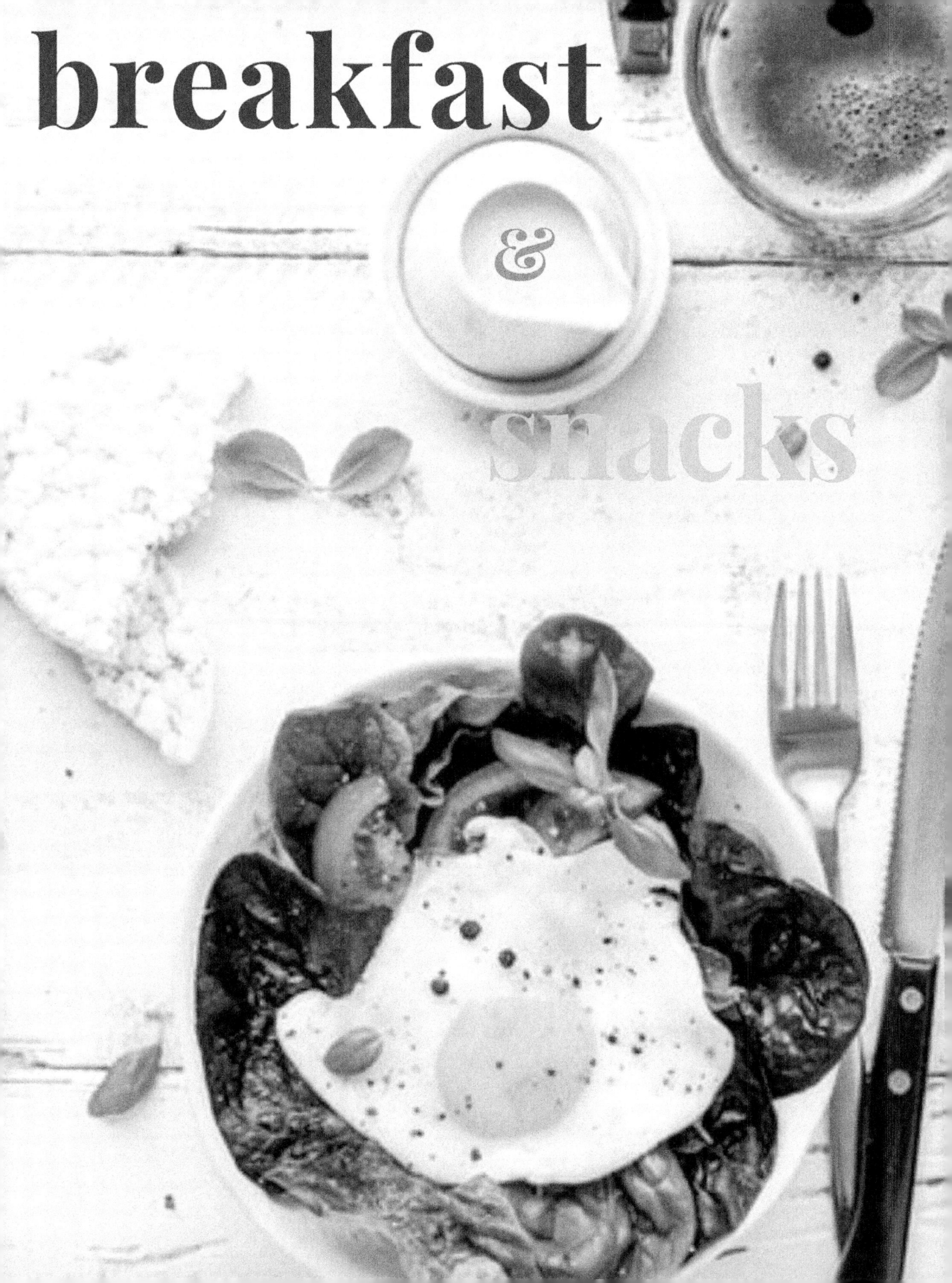

Breakfast and Snacks

1. Bacon and Avocado Omelet

Preparation time: 5 minutes

Cooking time: 5 minutes

Servings: 1

Ingredients:

- 1 slice of crispy bacon
- 2 organic eggs
- 1/2 cup grated parmesan cheese
- 2 tbsp. Ghee
- 1 avocado

Nutrition:

- Calories: 719
- Carbohydrate: 3.3 g
- Fat: 63 g
- Protein: 30 g

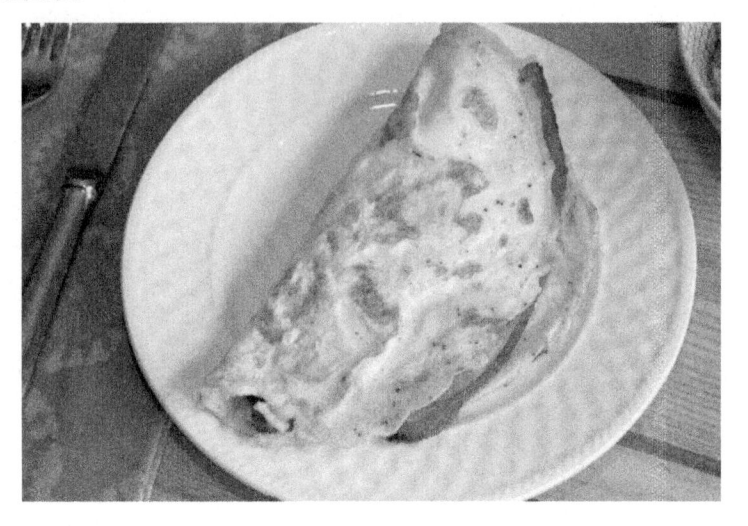

Directions:

1. Cook the bacon and set it aside.
2. Mix the eggs and parmesan cheese.
3. Heat a skillet and add the ghee to melt. Mix in the eggs, then cooks for 30 seconds.
4. Flip and cook again for 30 seconds.
5. Serve with the crunched bacon bits and sliced avocado.

2. Keto Smoked Salmon with Avocado Slice

Preparation time: 10 mins

Cooking time: 5 minutes

Servings: 2

Ingredients:

- 1/2 avocado
- 1 tsp. lemon juice
- 2 tsp. capers
- 1 tsp. chopped cilantro
- A pinch crushed red pepper flake
- 2 slices of smoked salmon
- Olive oil to taste
- Salt to taste

Nutrition:

- Calories: 212
- Fat: 11 g
- Carbohydrates: 10 g
- Fiber: 5 g
- Sugar: 2 g
- Protein: 15.6 g

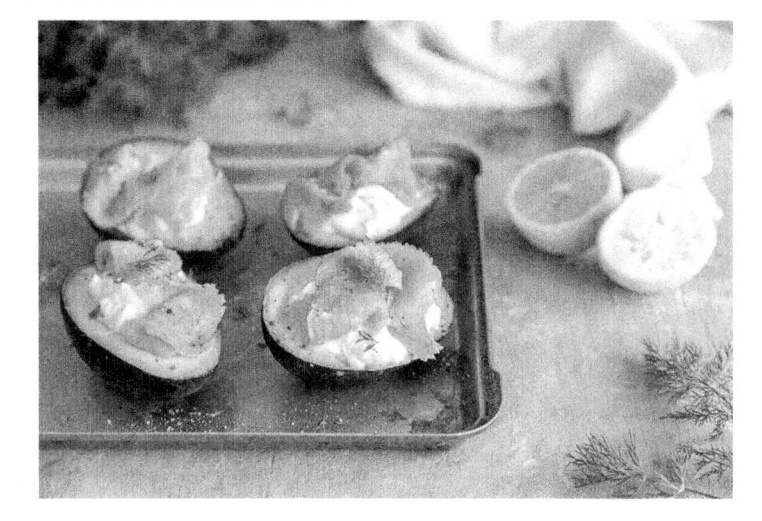

Directions:

1. Scoop the avocado from its skin and place it in a bowl. Add the lemon juice, capers, cilantro, red pepper flakes, olive oil, and salt, and mix well. Slice the salmon into two long strips. Place one of them on each plate. Divide the avocado mixture between the plates or serve on top.

3. Keto Cereal with Almond Milk and Walnuts

Preparation time: 5 minutes

Cooking time: 2 minutes

Servings: 2

Ingredients:

- 1/3 cup old-fashioned oatmeal
- 1/2 cup unsweetened vanilla almond milk
- 2 tbsp. chopped walnuts
- **Suggested additions:** Vanilla extract, cinnamon, or any other flavorings of choice

Directions:

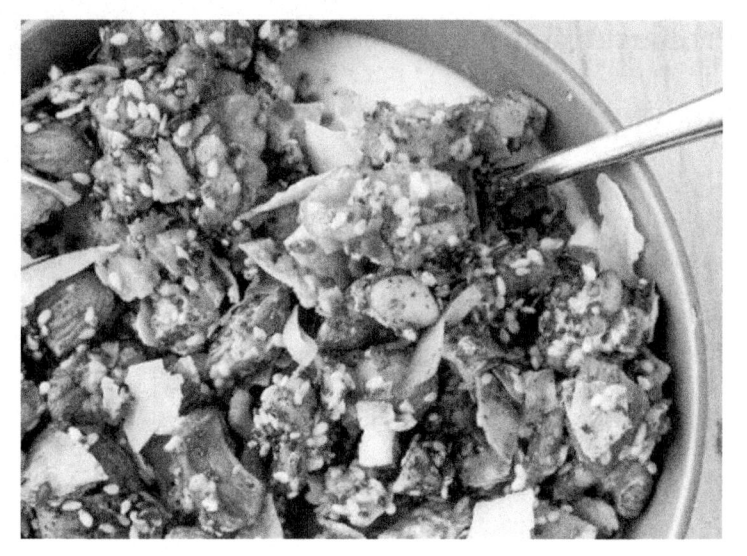

1. Using your hands, mix the oatmeal with the almond milk and walnuts.
2. Form into a bowl and serve with your favorite toppings, such as additional nuts, strawberries, or blueberries.

Nutrition:

- Calories: 38
- Fat: 1 g
- Carbohydrates: 2 g
- Fiber: 1 g
- Sugar: 0 g
- Protein: 3 g

4. Kale Fritters

Preparation time: 5 minutes

Cooking time: 4 minutes

Servings: 6

Ingredients:

- 7 oz. kale, chopped (tiny pieces)
- 10 oz. zucchini, washed and grated
- 1 tsp. basil
- 1/2 tsp. salt
- 1/4 cup almond flour
- 1/2 tbsp. mustard
- 1 large egg
- 1 tbsp. coconut milk
- 1 white onion, diced
- 1 tbsp. olive oil

Nutrition:

- Calories: 110
- Carbohydrates: 4 g
- Fat: 5 g
- Protein: 16 g

Directions:

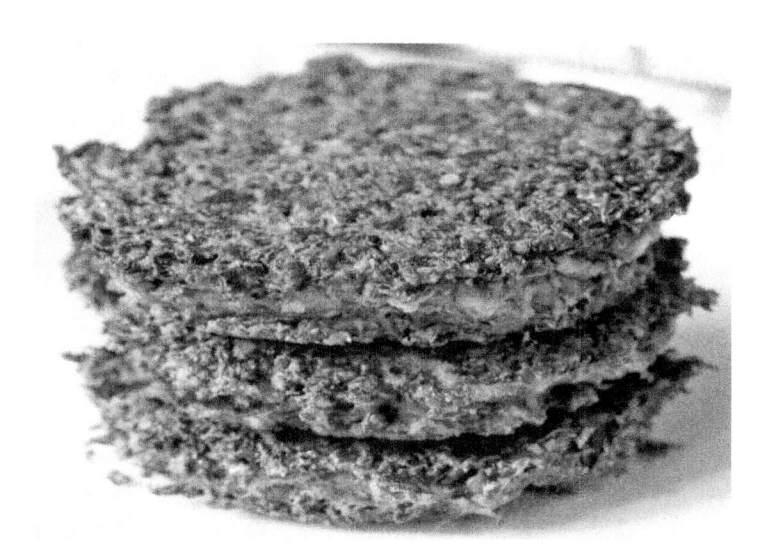

1. In a medium bowl, mix kale and zucchini. Add basil and salt and stir. Add almond flour and mustard. Stir well.
2. In another bowl, whisk together egg, coconut milk, and onion. Pour egg mixture into zucchini mixture and knead the thick dough.
3. Preheat the pan with olive oil on medium heat. Shape fritters with the help of a spoon and put them in the pan. Cook fritters for about 2 minutes per side. Transfer fritters to a paper towel to remove excess oil. Serve hot.

5. Cream Cheese Eggs

Preparation time: 5 minutes

Cooking time: 5 minutes

Servings: 1

Ingredients:

- 1 tbsp. butter
- 2 eggs
- 2 tbsp. soft cream cheese with chives

Nutrition:

- Calories: 341
- Carbohydrates: 3 g
- Fat: 31 g
- Protein: 15 g

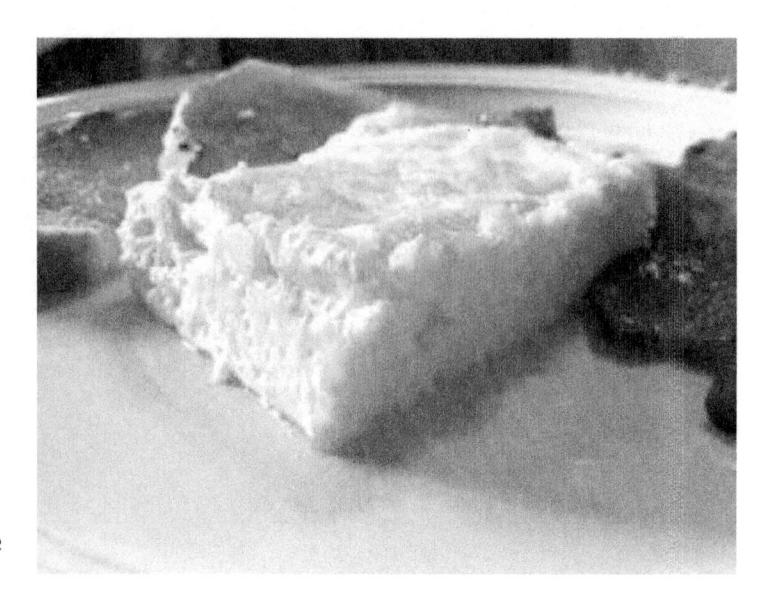

Directions:

1. Heat a skillet and melt the butter. Whisk the eggs with the cream cheese.
2. Cook until done. Serve.

6. Creamy Basil Baked Sausage

Preparation time: 5 minutes

Cooking time: 5 minutes

Servings: 12

Ingredients:

- 3 lb. Italian sausage
- 8 oz. cream cheese
- 25 cup heavy cream
- 1/4 cup basil pesto
- 8 oz. mozzarella

Nutrition:

- Calories: 316
- Carbohydrates: 4 g
- Fat: 23 g
- Protein: 23 g

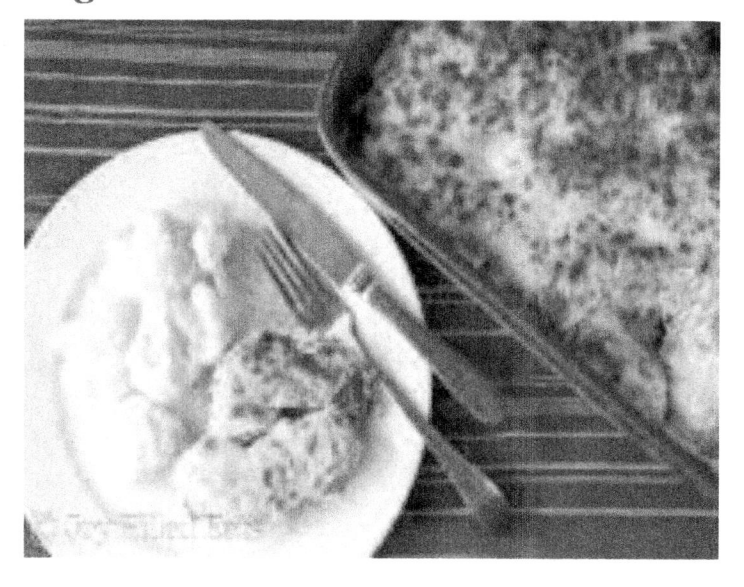

Directions:

1. Set the oven at 400°F.
2. Put the sausage in the dish and bake for 30 minutes. Combine the heavy cream, pesto, and cream cheese. Pour the sauce over the casserole and top it off with the cheese.
3. Bake for 10 minutes. Serve.

7. Almond Coconut Egg Wraps

Preparation time: 5 minutes

Cooking time: 5 minutes

Servings: 4

Ingredients:

- 5 organic eggs
- 1 tbsp. coconut flour
- 1/4 tsp. sea salt
- 2 tbsp. almond meal

Nutrition:

- Calories: 111
- Carbohydrates: 3 g
- Fat: 8 g
- Protein: 8 g

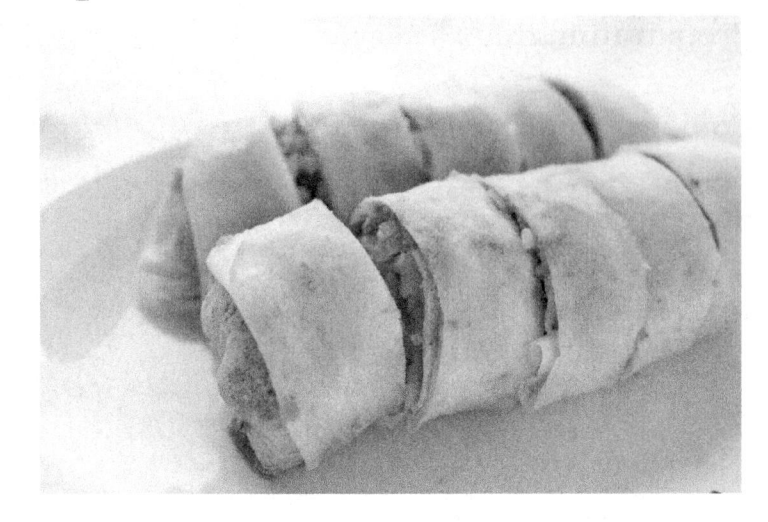

Directions:

1. Blend the ingredients in a blender. Warm-up a skillet, medium-high.
2. Put 2 tablespoons of the mixture then cook for 3 minutes.
3. Flip to cook for another 3 minutes. Serve.

8. Ricotta Cloud Pancakes

Preparation time: 5 minutes

Cooking time: 2 minutes

Servings: 4

Ingredients:

- 1 cup almond flour
- 1 tsp. low carb baking powder
- 2 1/2 tbsp. swerve
- 1/3 tsp. salt
- 1 1/4 cup ricotta cheese
- 1/3 cup coconut milk
- 2 large eggs
- 1 cup heavy whipping cream

Nutrition:

- Calories: 407
- Carbohydrates: 7 g
- Fat: 31 g
- Protein: 12 g

Directions:

1. In a medium bowl, whisk the almond flour, baking powder, swerve, and salt. Set aside.
2. Then, crack the eggs into the blender and process them at medium speed for 30 seconds. Add the ricotta cheese, continue processing it, and gradually pour the coconut milk in while you keep on blending.
3. In about 90 seconds, the mixture will be creamy and smooth. Pour it into the dry ingredients and whisk to combine.
4. Set a skillet over medium heat and let it heat for a minute. Then, fetch a soup spoonful of mixture into the skillet and cook it for 1 minute.
5. Flip the pancake and cook further for 1 minute. Remove onto a plate and repeat the cooking process until the batter is xhausted. Serve the pancakes with whipping cream.

9. Keto Cinnamon Coffee

Preparation time: 5 minutes

Cooking time: 5 minutes

Servings: 1

Ingredients:

- 2 tbsp. ground coffee
- 1/3 cup heavy whipping cream
- 1 tsp. ground cinnamon
- 2 cups of water

Nutrition:

- Calories: 136
- Carbohydrates: 1 g
- Fiber: 1 g
- Fat: 14 g
- Protein: 1 g

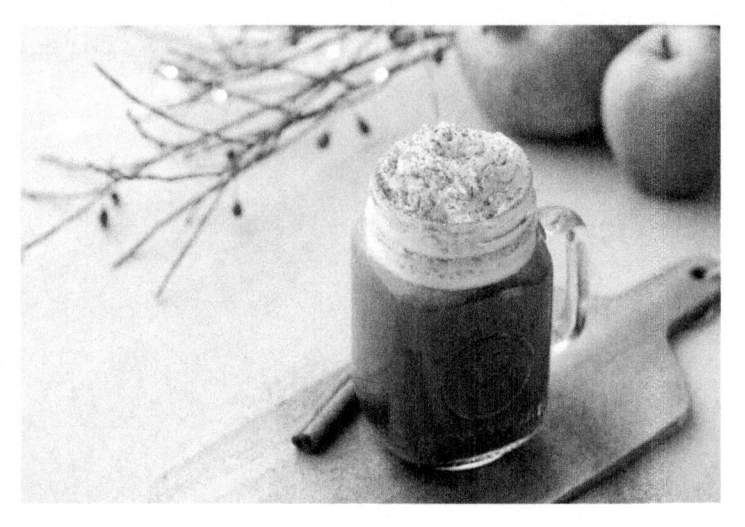

Directions:

1. Start by mixing the cinnamon with the ground coffee.
2. Pour in hot water, whip the cream until stiff peaks.
3. Serve with cinnamon.

10. Keto Coconut Flake Balls

Preparation time: 10 minutes

Cooking time: 0 minutes

Servings: 2

Ingredients:

- 1 vanilla shortbread collagen protein bar
- 1 tbsp. lemon
- 1/4 tsp. ground ginger
- 1/2 cup unsweetened coconut flakes
- 1/4 tsp. ground turmeric
- 1 spoon of water

Nutrition:

- Calories: 204
- Carbohydrates: 4.2 g
- Fat: 11 g
- Protein: 1.5 g

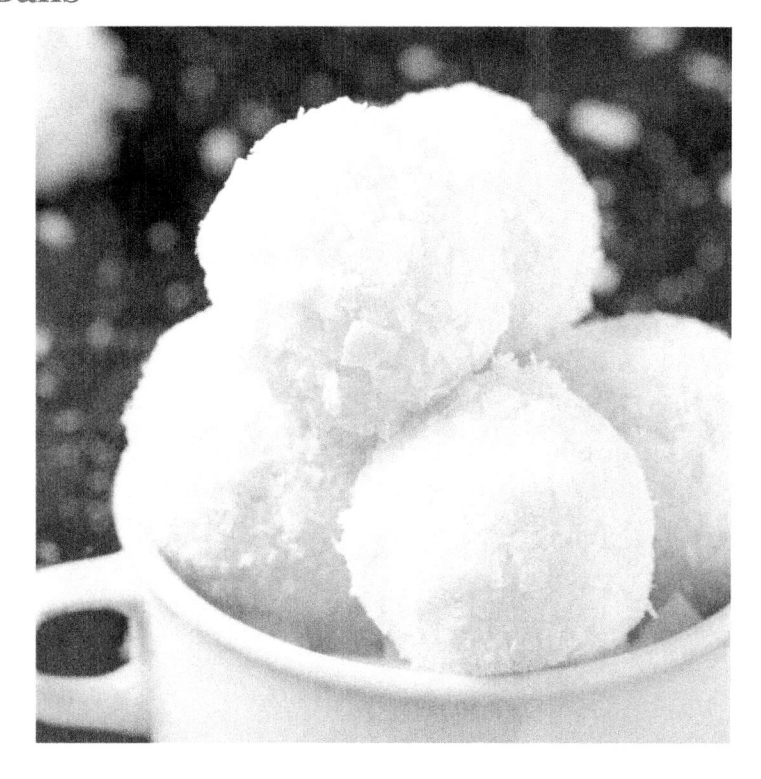

Directions:

1. Process protein bar, ginger, turmeric, and 3/4 of the total flakes into a food processor.
2. Remove and add 1 spoon of water and 1 tbsp. lemon and roll till dough forms.
3. Roll into balls and sprinkle the rest of the flakes on it. Serve.

11. Smoked Salmon and Poached Eggs on Toast

Preparation time: 5 Minutes

Cooking time: 4 Minutes

Servings: 4

Ingredients:

- 2 oz. avocado smashed
- 2 slices of bread toasted
- A pinch of kosher salt and cracked black pepper
- 1/4 tsp. freshly squeezed lemon juice
- 2 eggs see notes, poached
- 3 1/2 oz. smoked salmon
- 1 tbsp. thinly sliced scallions
- Splash of Kikkoman soy sauce (optional)
- Microgreens are (optional)

Nutrition:

- Calories: 459
- Fat: 22 g
- Carbohydrates: 33 g
- Protein: 31 g

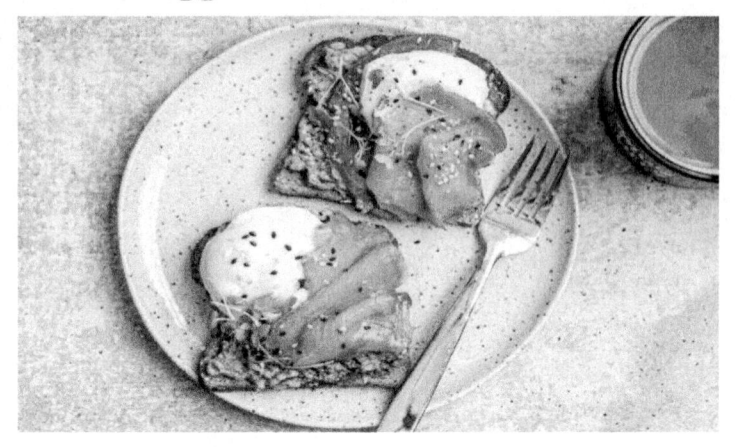

Directions:

1. Take a small bowl and then smash the avocado into it. Then, add the lemon juice and a pinch of salt into the mixture. Then, mix it well and set it aside.
2. After that, poach the eggs and toast the bread for some time.
3. Once the bread is toasted, you will have to spread the avocado on both slices and after that, add the smoked salmon to each slice.
4. Thereafter, carefully transfer the poached eggs to the respective toasts.
5. Add a splash of Kikkoman soy sauce and some cracked pepper; then, just garnish with scallions and microgreens.

12. Chocolate Banana Smoothie

Smoothies are great for breakfast on the go because they are quick, fill you up, and provide lasting energy throughout the morning.

Preparation time: 10 mins

Cooking time: 0 minutes

Servings: 2

Ingredients:

- 2 bananas, peeled
- 1 cup unsweetened almond milk, or skim milk
- 1 cup crushed ice
- 3 tbsp. unsweetened cocoa powder
- 3 tbsp. honey

Nutrition:

- Calories: 246
- Carbohydrates: 24.5 g
- Fat: 11.1 g
- Fiber: 4.7 g
- Protein: 13.7 g

Directions:

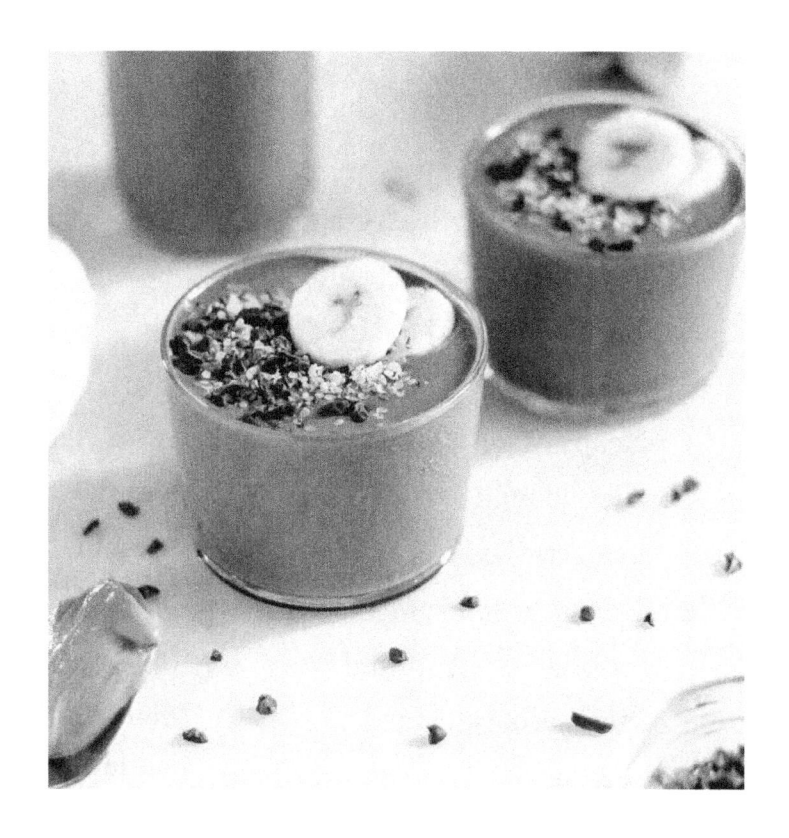

1. In a blender, combine the bananas, almond milk, ice, cocoa powder, and honey.
2. Blend until smooth.
3. You can refrigerate leftovers and blend the next day for about 30 seconds at high speed.

13. Fruit Smoothie

Preparation time: 5 minutes

Cooking time: 5 minutes

Servings: 2

Ingredients:

- 2 cups blueberries (or any fresh or frozen fruit, cut into pieces if the fruit is large)
- 2 cups unsweetened almond milk
- 1 cup crushed ice
- 1/2 tsp. ground ginger (or other dried ground spice such as turmeric, cinnamon, or nutmeg)

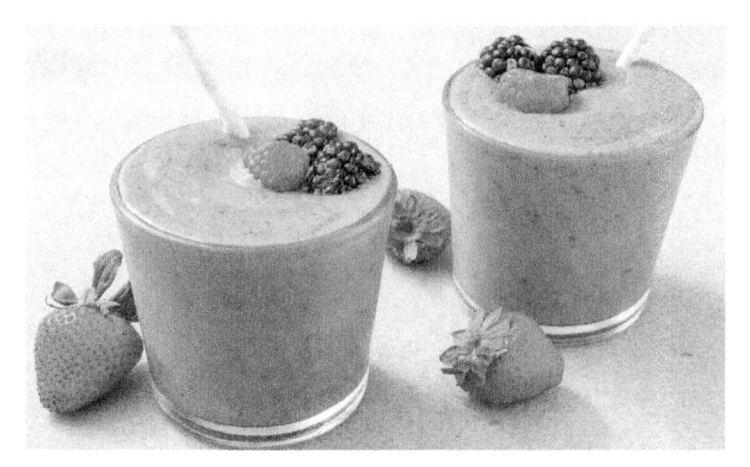

Directions:

1. In a blender, combine the blueberries, almond milk, ice, and ginger. Blend until smooth.
2. Some flavor combinations to try ginger and blueberry, honeydew melon and turmeric, mango and nutmeg, or mixed berries and cinnamon. Have fun experimenting

Note:

The great thing about fruit smoothies is how easy it is to customize them using seasonal produce. Because fruit is naturally sweet, you don't need to add any additional sweetener here. If using seasonal fruits, opt for fresh. In the absence of seasonal fruits, use frozen fruits.

Nutrition:

- Calories: 246
- Carbohydrates: 24.5 g
- Fat: 11.1 g
- Fiber: 4.7 g
- Protein: 13.7 g

14. Berry Smoothie

Preparation time: 10 minutes

Cooking time: 0 minutes

Servings: 2

Ingredients:

- 1/2 cup vanilla low-fat Greek yogurt
- 1/4 cup low-fat milk
- 1/2 cup fresh or frozen blueberries or strawberries (or a combination)
- 6–8 ice cubes

Nutrition:

- Calories: 90
- Carbohydrates: 23.9 g
- Fat: 0.3 g
- Protein: 0.5 g

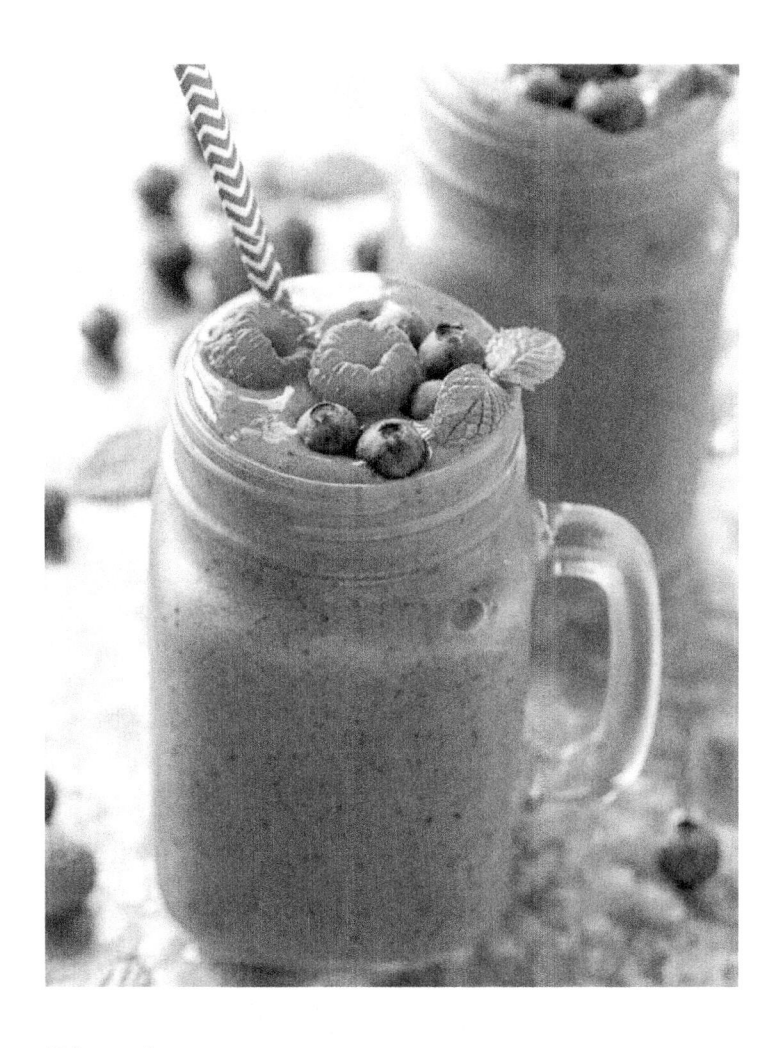

Directions:

1. Place the Greek yogurt, milk, and berries in a blender and blend until the berries are liquefied. Add the ice cubes and blend on high until thick and smooth. Serve immediately.

15. Strawberry Rhubarb Smoothie

Preparation time: 8 minutes

Cooking time: 0 minutes

Servings: 2

Ingredients:

- 1 cup strawberries, fresh and sliced
- 1 rhubarb stalk, chopped
- 2 tbsp. honey, raw
- 3 ice cubes
- 1/8 tsp. ground cinnamon
- 1/2 cup Greek yogurt, plain
- Water

Nutrition:

- Calories: 295
- Fat: 8 g
- Carbohydrates: 56 g
- Protein: 6 g

Directions:

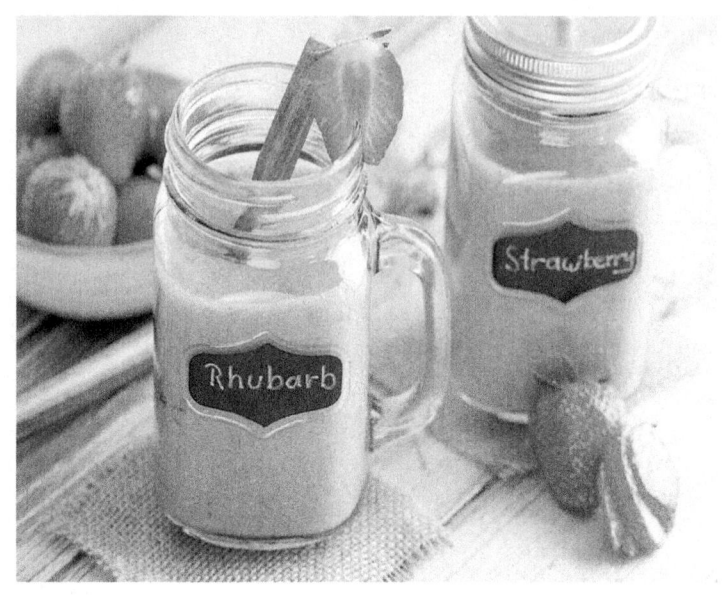

1. Start by getting out a small saucepan and fill it with water. Place it over high heat to bring it to a boil, and then add in your rhubarb.
2. Boil for 3 minutes before draining and transferring it to a blender.
3. In your blender, add in your yogurt, honey, cinnamon, and strawberries. Blend until smooth, and then add in your ice.
4. Blend until there are no lumps and it's thick. Enjoy cold.

lunch & dinner

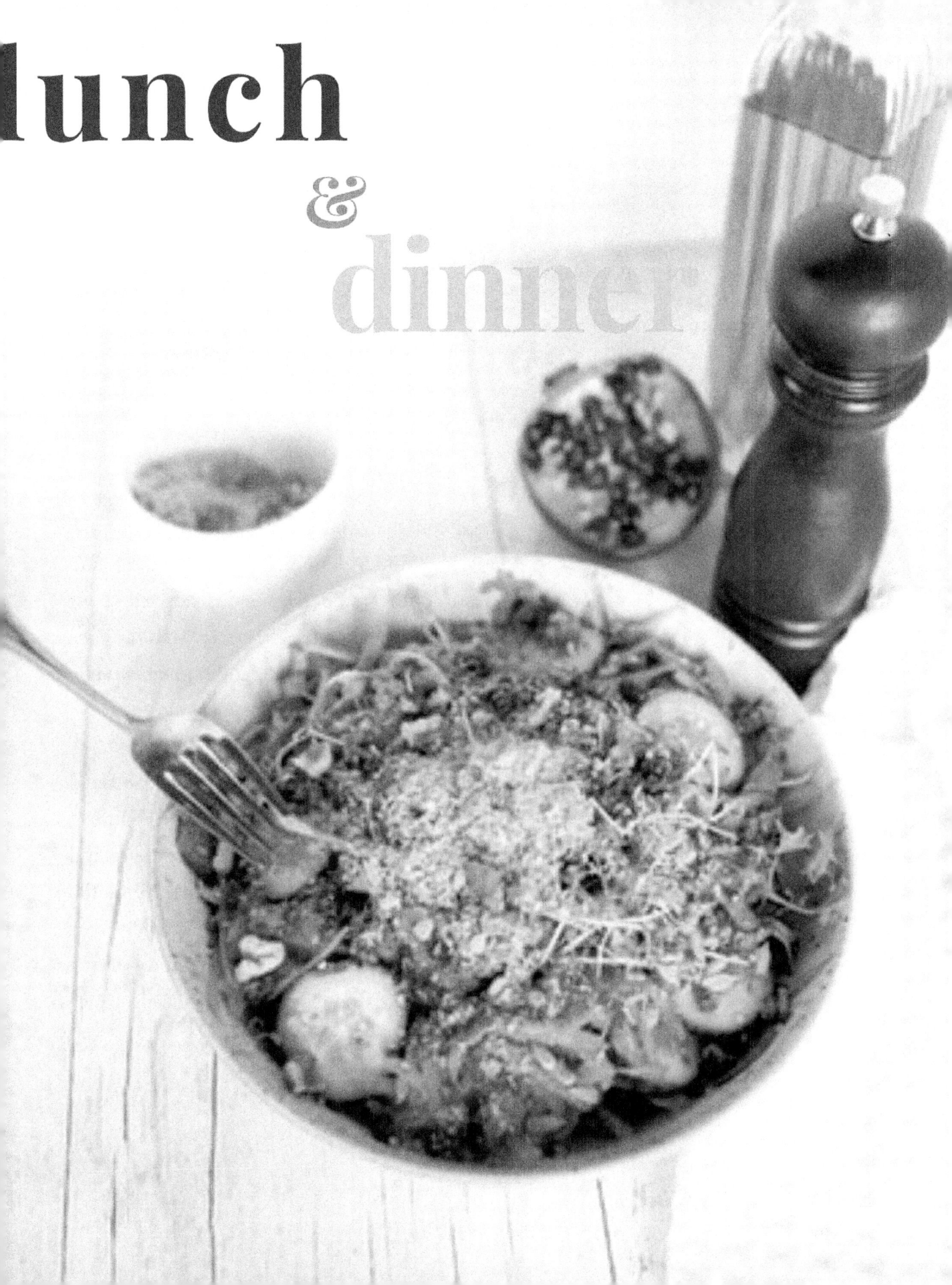

Lunch and Dinner Recipes

16. Cilantro Chicken Breasts with Mayo-Avocado Sauce

Preparation time: 5 minutes

Cooking time: 20 minutes

Servings: 4

Ingredients:

Mayo-avocado sauce:

- 1 avocado, pitted
- 1/2 cup mayonnaise
- Salt to taste

Chicken:

- 2 tbsp. ghee
- 4 chicken breasts
- Pink salt and black pepper to taste
- 2 tbsp. fresh cilantro, chopped
- 1/2 cup chicken broth

Nutrition:

- Calories: 398
- Fat: 32 g
- Carbohydrates: 4 g
- Protein 24 g

Directions:

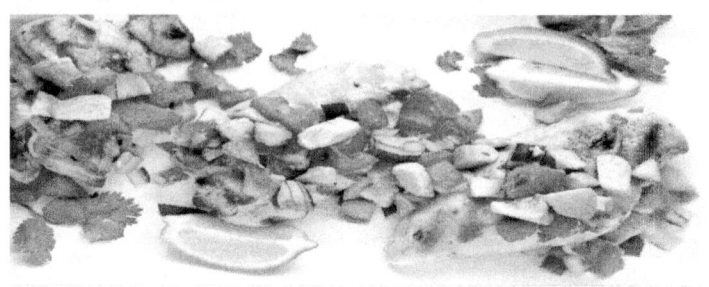

1. Spoon the avocado into a bowl and mash with a fork. Add in mayonnaise and salt and stir until a smooth sauce is derived. Pour sauce into a jar and refrigerate. Melt the ghee in a large skillet over medium heat. Season chicken with salt and pepper and fry for 4 minutes on each side until golden brown.
2. Pour the broth in the same skillet and add the cilantro. Bring to simmer covered for 3 minutes and return the chicken. Cover and cook on low heat for 5 minutes until the liquid has reduced and the chicken is fragrant. Place the chicken only into serving plates and spoon the mayo-avocado sauce over. Serve.

17. Sweet Garlic Chicken Skewers

Preparation time: 10 Mins

Cooking time: 15 Minutes

Servings: 4

Ingredients:

Skewers:

- 3 tbsp. soy sauce
- 1 tbsp. ginger-garlic paste
- 2 tbsp. swerve brown sugar
- 1 tsp. chili pepper
- 2 tbsp. olive oil
- 1 lb. chicken breasts, cut into cubes

Dressing

- 1/2 cup tahini
- 1/2 tsp. garlic powder
- Pink salt to taste
- 1/4 cup of warm water

Nutrition:

- Calories: 225
- Fat: 17.4 g
- Carbohydrates: 2 g
- Protein: 15 g

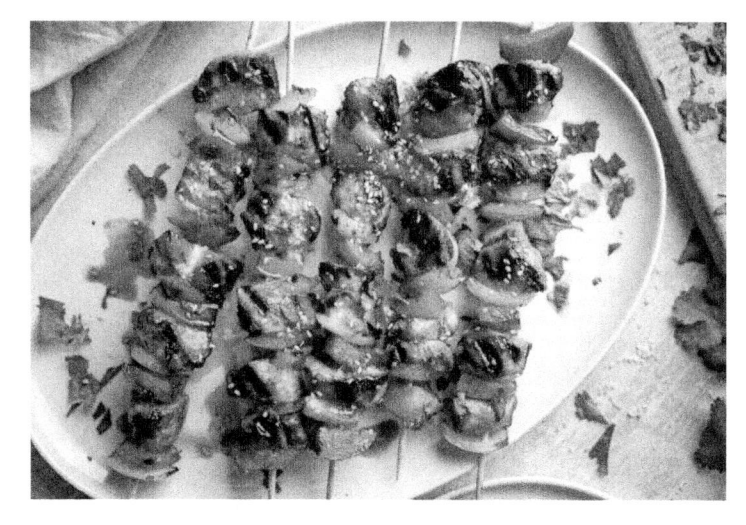

Directions:

1. In a bowl, whisk soy sauce, ginger-garlic paste, swerve brown sugar, chili pepper, and olive oil. Put the chicken in a zipper bag. Pour in the marinade, seal, and shake to coat. Marinate in the fridge for 2 hours.
2. Preheat grill to 400°F. Thread the chicken on skewers. Cook for 10 minutes in total with three to four turnings until golden brown; remove to a plate. Mix the tahini, garlic powder, salt, and 1/4 cup of warm water in a bowl. Pour into serving jars. Serve the chicken skewers and tahini dressing with Cauli rice.

18. Keto Chinese Pork Stew with Cabbage

Preparation time: 15 minutes

Cooking time: 30 minutes

Servings: 2

Ingredients:

- 1 tbsp. peanut oil or avocado oil, divided
- 4 oz. bacon, sliced thickly
- 1/2 cup red cabbage, finely shredded
- 2 garlic cloves, minced
- 1 tbsp. grated fresh ginger root
- 1/4 tsp. crushed red pepper flakes, or to taste (optional)
- 2 tsp. dark sesame oil, divided
- 1/4 cup coconut Aminos or low sodium soy sauce

Nutrition:

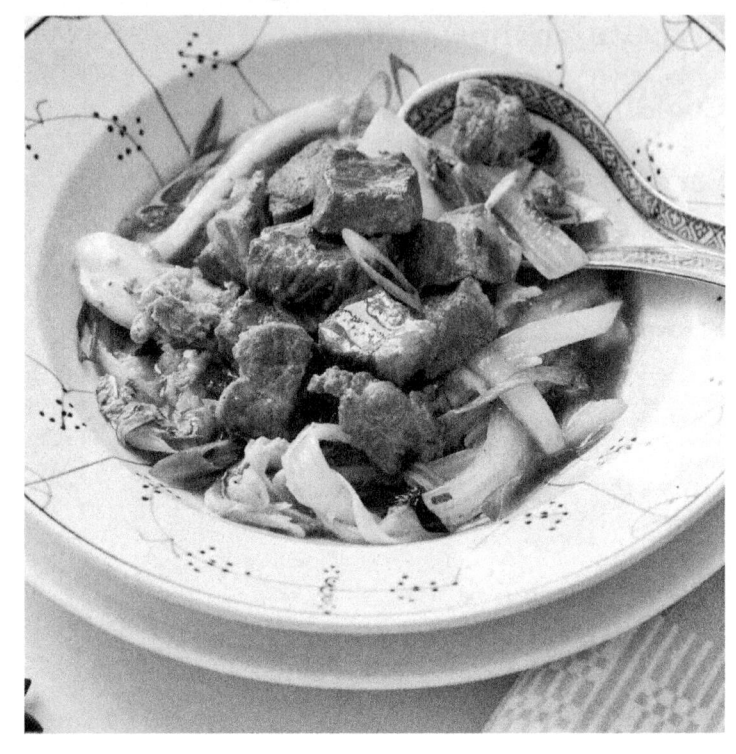

Directions:

1. Heat 1 tsp. peanut oil in a large, deep skillet over high heat. Add the bacon and cook until crispy. Transfer to a bowl and set aside.
2. Add the remaining oil to the skillet and then add half the red cabbage. Cook, stirring often, until wilted-about 3 minutes, then transfer to a large bowl.
3. Add the garlic, ginger root, and red pepper flakes to the skillet; cook 1 minute over medium-low heat. Stir in half the sesame oil

- Calories: 76
- Fat: 5 g
- Carbohydrates: 3 g
- Fiber: 1 g
- Sugar: 0 g
- Protein: 5 g

and stir in enough of the bacon drippings or other fat to coat the pan. Cook 3 minutes over medium-low heat for a slightly thickened sauce.

4. Stir in the cabbage, bacon, coconut Aminos, and soy sauce. Cook until the cabbage is heated through, and the sauce has thickened about 7 minutes. This should be done over low heat, so you don't overcook the cabbage. Transfer to a serving bowl and sprinkle with remaining sesame oil before serving with steamed white rice or your favorite grain.

19. Keto Zucchini Lasagna

Preparation time: 15 mins

Cooking time: 45 minutes

Servings: 2

Ingredients:

- 16 oz. ricotta cheese, divided
- 1 tbsp. dried Italian seasoning, divided
- 2 tbsp. grated Parmesan cheese, divided
- 2/3 cup low-fat cottage cheese
- 1 large egg plus 3 egg whites, lightly beaten (or 2 whole eggs)
- 5 cups chopped zucchini
- 1 1/2 cups jarred tomato sauce
- 2 cups shredded mozzarella cheese, divided
- Cooking spray

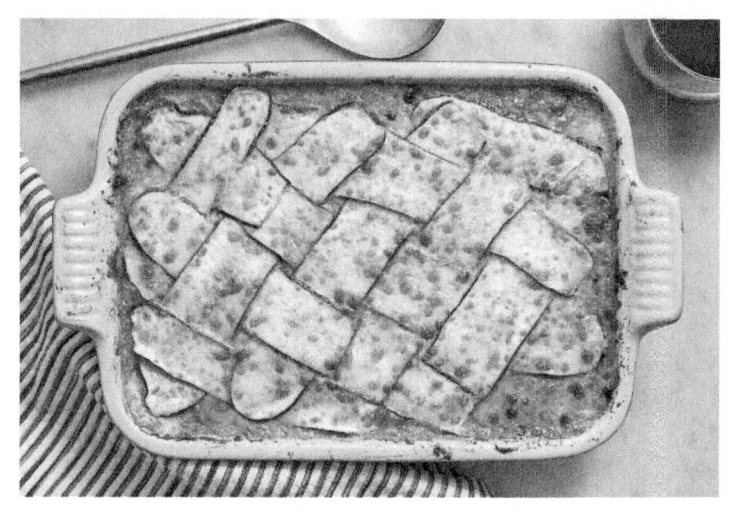

Directions:

1. Preheat oven to 400°F. Coat a 9-by-13-inch baking dish with nonstick cooking spray. Set aside. In a medium bowl, stir together 1/3 cup of the ricotta cheese, 1 tsp. of Italian seasoning, and 1 tsp. of Parmesan cheese; set aside. In another bowl, combine cottage cheese, egg, and egg whites, season with salt and pepper if desired. To make the lasagna rolls, layout flat about 5 sheets of lasagna noodles (3 to 4 inches wide) at a time on your countertop. Spoon about a quarter of the cottage cheese mixture in a line down the middle of the lasagna sheets, being careful not to spread it out. Sprinkle a small amount

- Salt and pepper to taste
- 5 sheets of lasagna noodles

Nutrition:

- Calories: 208
- Fat: 10.6 g
- Carbohydrates: 12.1 g
- Fiber: 2.3 g
- Sugar: 4.7 g
- Protein: 16.2 g

of mozzarella cheese, zucchini, and tomato sauce over the cottage cheese mixture. Then evenly lay out more lasagna sheets on top of this (about 5 or 6 sheets) and fold over the ends to cover it.

2. Roll up the lasagna sheet with the cottage cheese mixture in it like you would roll up a jelly roll and transfer it to an ungreased baking dish seam side down. Repeat for all remaining ingredients to create 3 more rolls in total. Cover the baking dish with aluminum foil and bake at 400°F for 45 minutes. Remove the foil and cover the dish again for 15 more minutes. Transfer to a serving plate, slice into 6 portions and sprinkle with remaining leftover Parmesan cheese.

20. Garlic Steak Bite Salad with Tarragon Dressing

Preparation time: 10 mins

Cooking time: 15 minutes

Servings: 2

Ingredients:

- 12 oz. flank steak, cut into bite-sized pieces
- 6 tbsp. butter, divided
- 4 garlic cloves, minced, divided
- 1 tsp. paprika, divided
- 3 cups baby arugula or spinach salad mix (about 1 oz.)
- 1 cup cherry tomatoes, halved or quartered if large
- 1/4 cup crumbled blue cheese (optional)
- Salt and pepper to taste

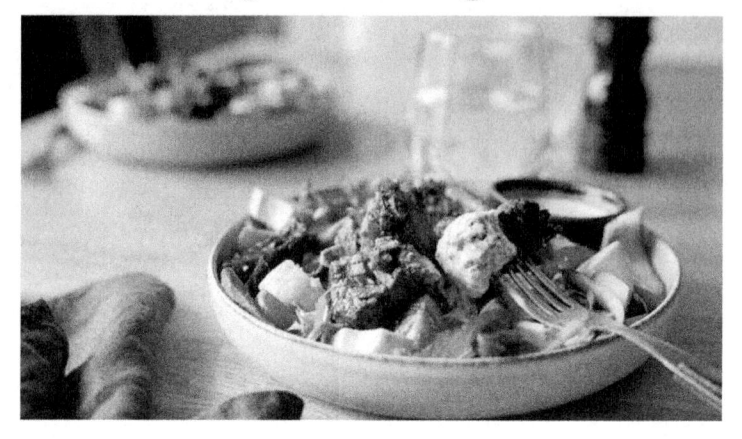

Directions:

1. In a small bowl add 1 tbsp. of the minced garlic and 2 tsp. paprika; set aside. Heat 2 tbsp. butter over medium-high heat in a large skillet for 30 seconds. Add the steak and season with salt and pepper; cook 6 minutes, tossing frequently to brown evenly on both sides. Transfer the steak to a plate. Add the remaining 2 tbsp. butter and the remaining 4 garlic cloves to the pan; cook 1 minute over medium heat.
2. Add the steak back into the pan with any juices that have accumulated on the plate, season with salt and pepper if desired. Lower heat to medium-low and stir in garlic-paprika mixture, cooking for an additional minute until fragrant. Pour into a large bowl

Nutrition:

- Calories: 214
- Fat: 15 g
- Carbohydrates: 3 g
- Fiber: 2 g
- Sugar: 0.5 g
- Protein: 15.5 g

and add arugula or spinach, tomatoes, and blue cheese if using. Toss until combined. Serve immediately or refrigerate for later use as it tastes best when eaten cold.

21. Keto Harvest Pumpkin and Sausage Soup

Preparation time: 15 mis

Cooking time: 20-30 mins

Servings: 2

Ingredients:

- 1 tsp. coconut oil, divided
- 1 lb. ground pork sausage (80/20)
- 1/2 tsp. ground nutmeg, divided
- 1 small onion, diced small (about 1/4 cup)
- 4 cups pumpkin puree (canned or fresh)
- 4 cups chicken broth
- 1 cup heavy whipping cream or coconut milk
- 2 tbsp. fresh sage, minced
- Salt and freshly ground black pepper to taste

Nutrition:

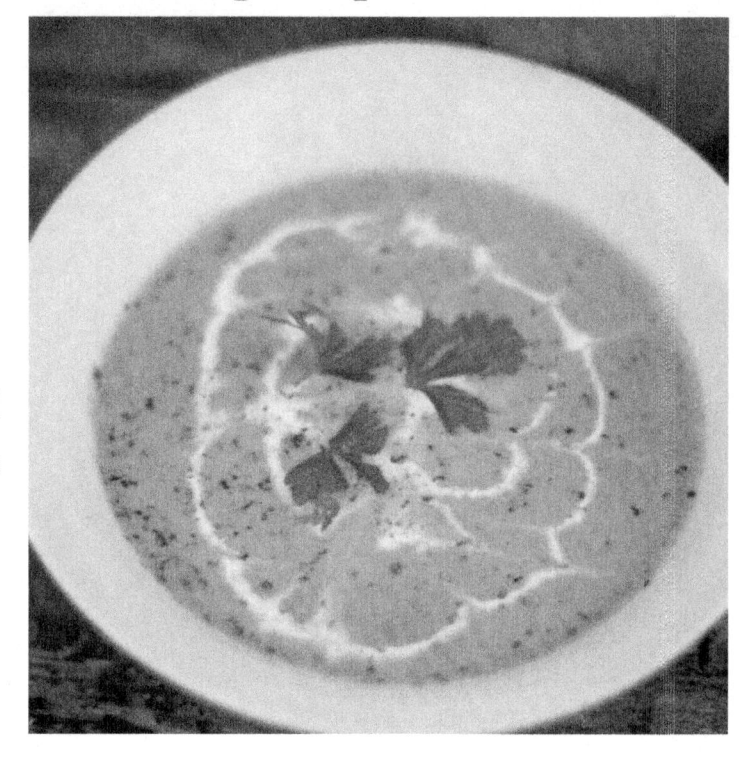

Directions:

1. Heat 1 tsp. of the oil in a medium saucepan over medium-high heat and add the sausage. Cook until well browned, stirring occasionally for about 10 minutes. Transfer sausage to a plate with a slotted spoon and set aside. Add the nutmeg to the sausage drippings in the saucepan; cook over low heat for 1 minute until fragrant, stirring constantly. Add the onion and cook 6

- Calories: 116
- Fat: 4 g
- Carbohydrates: 6.5 g
- Fiber: 2.6 g
- Sugar: 3 g
- Protein: 12.7 g

minutes until translucent, stirring frequently.

2. Add the remaining 1 tsp. oil to the saucepan; stir in pumpkin, broth, and cream, and bring to a simmer. Simmer for 4 minutes, stirring occasionally. Add the browned sausage with any juices back into the pot and stir well until well blended. Place mixture in a blender or food processor and blend until smooth, adding a little water, if needed. Stir in sage, salt and pepper then place back into the saucepan over medium heat; cook for 5 to 10 minutes until warm.

22. Keto Pulled Pork with Roasted Tomato Salad

Preparation time: 15 mins

Cooking time: 50 to 60 mins

Servings: 2

Ingredients:

- 1 small yellow onion, chopped
- 2 garlic cloves, minced
- 1 tbsp. olive oil
- 3/4 cup chicken broth or water (or more if needed)
- 4 cups fresh baby spinach
- 2 Tomatoes
- Salt and pepper to taste
- 3 lb. pork shoulder

Nutrition:

- Calories: 438
- Fat: 28 g
- Carbohydrates: 2.4 g
- Fiber: 0.4 g

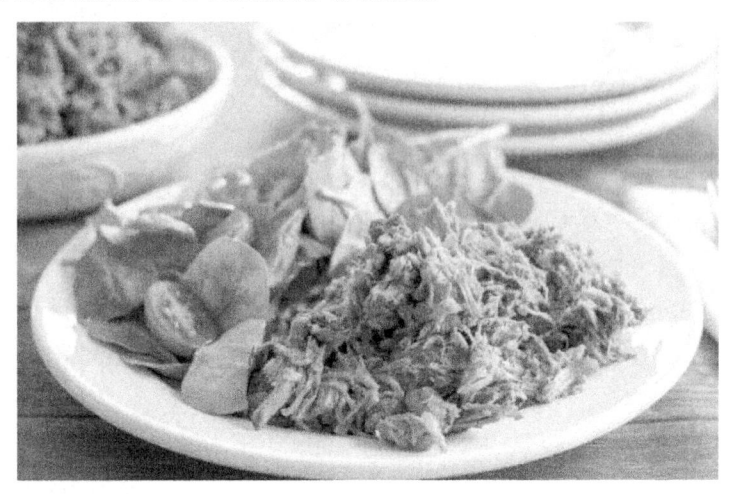

Directions:

1. Heat oven to 425°F. Wash the tomatoes. Cut the tops off and slice them in half lengthwise. Remove the seeds and sprinkle with salt and pepper. Put on a baking sheet and drizzle with olive oil, then roast for 20 minutes until soft. Using the same pan from roasting tomatoes, add olive oil over medium-high heat in a large skillet. Add whichever protein you choose into your skillet (in this recipe, I used a 3 lb. pork shoulder roast). Cook until browned evenly, breaking up the meat with a wooden spoon. Add 1 chopped onion into the skillet and cook for 4 to 5 minutes. Add the garlic and broth/water; reduce heat to low and simmer for another 6 to 8 minutes

- Sugar: 0.5 g
- Protein: 51.5 g

or until meat is cooked through. Transfer meat to a large bowl and set aside. In a large skillet, add remaining onions, spinach leaves and drizzle with olive oil. Season with salt and pepper if desired. Cook over medium heat for 2 to 3 minutes until wilted yet still bright green in color (adjust cooking time as needed). Serve the pulled pork with roasted tomatoes and spinach salad.

23. Thai Keto Tuna Salad Wrap

Preparation time: 15 mins

Cooking time: 15 to 20 mins

Servings: 2

Ingredients:

- 4 large collard green leaves, washed and blotted dry (2 heaping cups)
- 4 oz. cooked wild salmon (about 3/4 cup)
- 1/2 cup of chopped fresh cilantro
- 1/2 cup chopped fresh basil or mint or both
- 1/2 cup spinach
- 1/2 tsp. paprika, divided
- 1/4 tsp. crushed red chili pepper flakes, divided
- Salt and freshly ground black pepper to taste
- Juice of 1 lime (about 1 tbsp.)

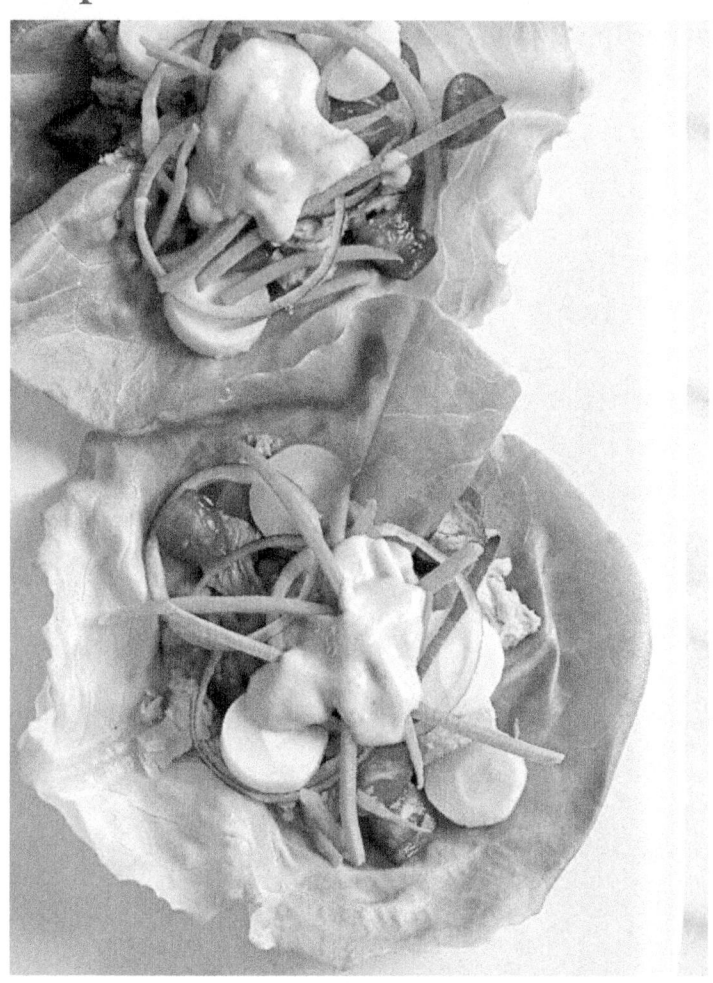

Directions:

1. Place a large skillet over medium-high heat. Add the olive oil into the skillet; swirl it around to coat. Add the tuna and season with salt, chili pepper, and paprika. Cook for about 3 minutes, tossing occasionally until

- 1 tbsp. olive oil or avocado oil (add more if needed)

Nutrition:

- Calories: 160
- Fat: 16 g
- Carbohydrates: 3 g
- Fiber: 1.5 g
- Sugar: 1 g
- Protein: 23.5 g

tuna is heated all the way through. Transfer tuna to a large bowl, then add spinach, basil or mint, cilantro, and lime juice to the bowl. Season with salt and pepper if desired. Toss until well blended then divide the mixture between the collard leaves; fold as needed to wrap them up. Serve with additional lime juice if desired. (Or shrimp or chicken for variation)

24. Chicken Bacon Burger

Preparation time: 10 Mins

Cooking time: 15 Mins

Servings: 8

Ingredients:

- 4 chicken breasts
- 4 slices of bacon
- 1/4 medium onion
- 2 garlic cloves
- 1/4 cup (60 ml) avocado oil, to cook with

Nutrition:

- Calories: 319
- Fat: 24 g
- Carbohydrates: 1 g
- Protein: 25 g

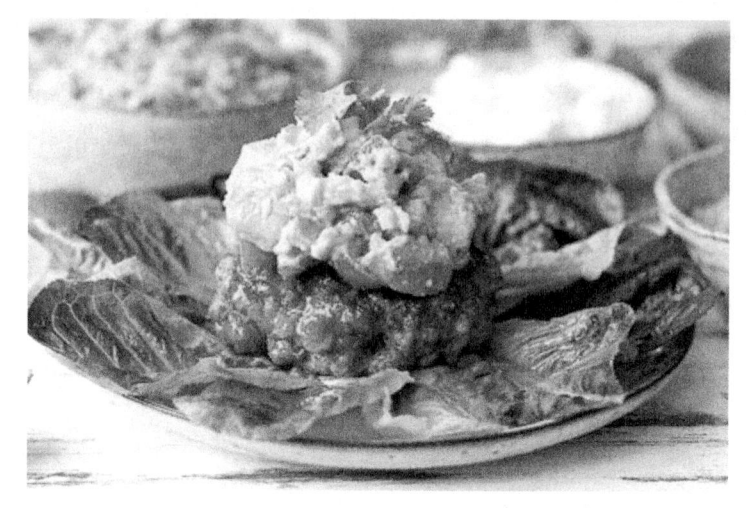

Directions:

1. Food process the chicken, bacon, onion, and garlic and form 8 patties. You need to do this in batches.
2. Fry patties in the avocado oil in batches. Make sure burgers are fully cooked.
3. Serve with guacamole.

25. Herby Fishcakes with Zucchini Salad

Preparation time: 15 mins

Cooking time: 20 to 25 mins

Servings: 2

Ingredients:

- 1 lb. firm white fish fillets (salmon or cod work best)
- 1 tsp. salt, divided
- 1/2 tsp. freshly ground black pepper, divided
- 1 cup cooked quinoa
- 2 scallions, thinly sliced (about 1/3 cup)
- Salt and freshly ground black pepper to taste
- Cooking spray
- 1 zucchini
- Oil to taste

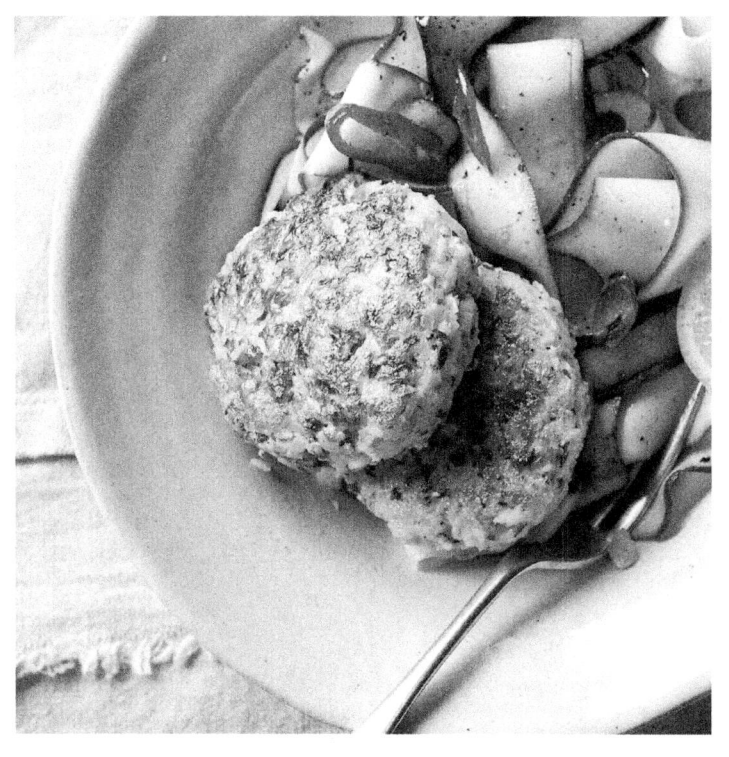

Directions:

1. Heat oven to 400°F then lines a baking sheet with parchment paper. Wash and pat dry the zucchini then cut into 1/4-inch-thick slices. Arrange slices in a single layer on the baking sheet then sprinkle with salt. Bake for 10 minutes until tender but still firm; set aside. Line a second baking sheet with aluminum foil and spray generously with nonstick cooking spray. Season the fish with 1 tsp. salt and 1/4 tsp. pepper. Heat a large skillet such

Nutrition:

- Calories: 135
- Fat: 4 g
- Carbohydrates: 6 g
- Fiber: 1.5 g
- Sugar: 0.5 g
- Protein: 17.5 g

as cast iron on medium heat and add enough oil to coat the bottom. Add the fish then cook for about 2 minutes, turning once. Transfer to the prepared baking sheet and continue with the remaining fish; cook in batches as needed.

2. Toast quinoa according to package directions and set aside until ready to use; set aside until "topping."
3. Heat broiler or grill (no oil required) and line a baking sheet with foil. Divide fish cakes between 4 bowls (about 1 1/2 tbsp. each); top each bowl with a spoonful of quinoa, zucchini than a sprinkle of scallions then remaining salt and pepper. Broil or grill fishcakes for 3 to 5 minutes until browned and heated through.

26. Lamb Burgers with Tzatziki

Preparation time: 10 Mins

Cooking time: 20 Minutes

Servings: 4

Ingredients:

- 1 lb. grass-fed lamb
- 1/4 cup chives finely chopped green onion or red onion if desired
- 1 tbsp. chopped fresh dill
- 1/2 tsp. dried oregano or about 1 tbsp. freshly chopped
- 1 tbsp. finely chopped fresh mint
- A pinch of chopped red pepper
- Fine-grained sea salt to taste
- 1 tbsp. water
- 2 tsp. olive oil to grease the pan

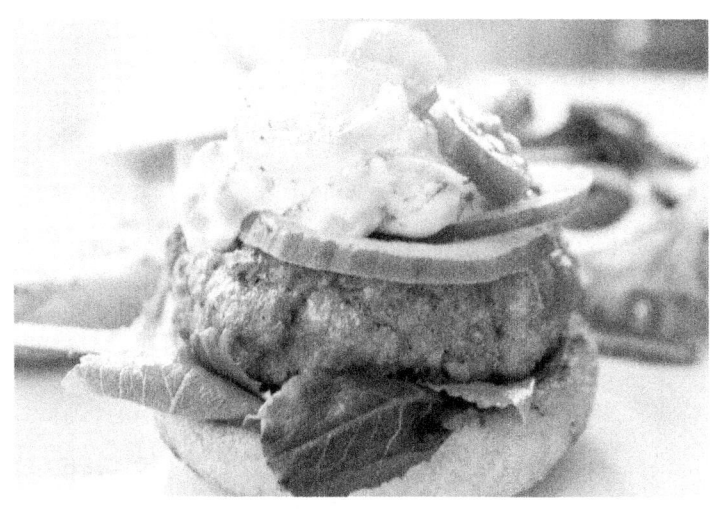

Directions:

1. Place the garlic, cucumber, and lemon juice in the food processor and press until finely chopped. Add the coconut cream, dill, salt, and pepper, and mix until well blended.
2. Put it in a jar with a lid and keep it in the refrigerator until it is served. The flavors become more intense over time when they cool in the fridge.
3. Thoroughly mix the ground lamb in a bowl with the chives or red onion, dill, oregano, mint, red pepper, and water.
4. Sprinkle the mixture with fine-grained sea salt and form 4 patties of the same size.

For the Tzatziki:

- 1 can coconut milk with all the cooled fat and 1 tbsp. the discarded liquid portion
- 3 garlic cloves
- 1 peeled cucumber without seeds, roughly sliced
- 1 tbsp. freshly squeezed lemon juice
- 2 tbsp. chopped fresh dill
- 3/4 tsp. fine grain sea salt
- Black pepper to taste

Nutrition:

- Calories: 363
- Fat: 22.14 g
- Carbohydrates: 6.83 g
- Protein: 35.33 g

5. Heat a large cast-iron skillet over medium heat and brush with a small amount of olive oil. Lightly sprinkle the pan with fine-grain sea salt.
6. Bring the patties into the pan and cook on each side for about 4 minutes, adjusting the heat to prevent the outside from becoming too brown. Alternatively, you can grill the burgers.
7. Remove from the pan and cover with Tzatziki sauce.

27. Lamb Sliders

Preparation time: 5 Minutes

Cooking time: 15 Minutes

Servings: 6

Ingredients:

- 1 lb. minced lamb or half veal, half lamb
- 1/2 sliced onion
- 2 garlic cloves minced
- 1 tbsp. dried dill
- 1 tsp. salt
- 1/2 tsp. black pepper

Nutrition:

- Calories: 207
- Fat: 11.89 g
- Carbohydrates: 1.17 g
- Protein: 22.68 g

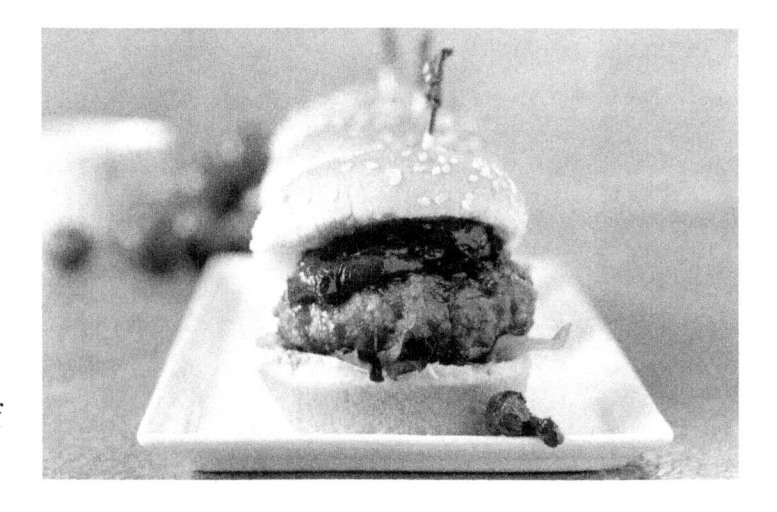

Directions:

1. Blend the ingredients gently in a large bowl until well combined. Overworking the meat will cause it to be tough.
2. Form the meat into burgers.
3. Grill or fry in a pan on medium-high heat until cooked through, 4 to 5 minutes per side. If preparing in a pan, sear both sides quickly, then throw the burgers in a 350°F oven for 10 minutes to finish cooking through.
4. Serve with Tzatziki for dipping!

28. Stuffed Keto Mushrooms

Preparation time: 10 minutes

Cooking time: 25 to 30 minutes

Servings: 2

Ingredients:

- 1 tbsp. butter or ghee
- 1/2 cup prepared cream cheese or full-fat mozzarella
- 1/4 tsp. salt, divided
- 1/4 tsp. freshly ground black pepper, divided
- 1/8 tsp. dried thyme, divided
- 4 oz. of your favorite ground meat (ground turkey or beef are good choices)
- 4 oz. Mushrooms

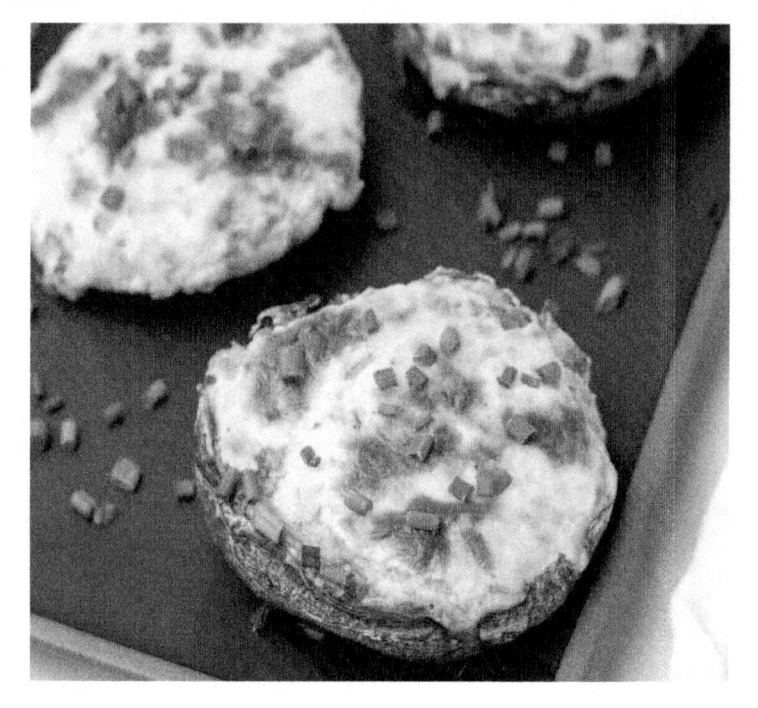

Directions:

1. Heat oven to 375°F. Melt butter/ghee in a small skillet over medium heat, then add mushrooms; sauté for 2 to 3 minutes. Add in the cream cheese, salt, pepper, and thyme; mix to combine. Stuff mushrooms with the mixture and transfer to a baking sheet lined with parchment paper, then drizzle with olive oil (if desired). Bake for 10 minutes until mushrooms are tender and cream cheese is softened; set aside.

Nutrition:

- Calories: 120
- Fat: 7 g
- Carbohydrates: 3 g
- Fiber: 0.5 g
- Sugar: 1 g
- Protein: 10 g

2. Heat a large skillet such as cast iron over medium heat then add the meat to the pan. Cook for about 5 minutes or until browned then season with remaining salt and pepper if desired.
3. Serve immediately with grilled vegetables or salad as desired. (Optional: top with additional mozzarella.)

29. Blackened Fish Tacos with Slaw

Preparation time: 14 Mins

Cooking time: 6 Minutes

Servings: 4

Ingredients:

- 1 tbsp. olive oil
- 1 tsp. chili powder
- 2 tilapia fillets
- 1 tsp. paprika
- 4 low carb tortillas

Slaw:

- 1/2 cup red cabbage, shredded
- 1 tbsp. lemon juice
- 1 tsp. apple cider vinegar
- 1 tbsp. olive oil
- Salt and black pepper to taste

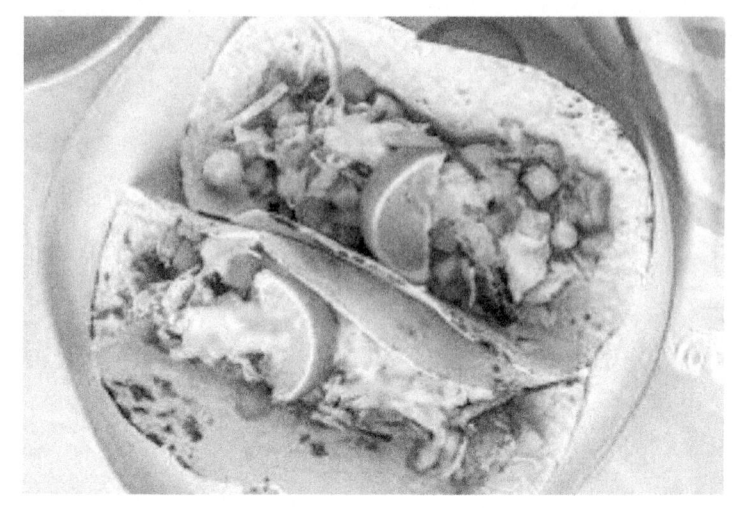

Directions:

1. Season the tilapia with chili powder and paprika. Heat the vegetable oil over a skillet over medium heat.
2. Add tilapia and cook until blackened, about 3 minutes per side. Cut into strips. Divide the tilapia between the tortillas. Blend all the slaw ingredients in a bowl and top the fish to serve.

Nutrition:

- Calories: 268
- Fat: 20 g
- Carbohydrates: 3.5 g
- Protein: 13.8 g

30. Zingy Lemon Fish

Preparation time: 10 mins

Cooking time: 15-20 minutes

Servings: 2

Ingredients:

- 1 tbsp. olive oil (optional)
- 2 tbsp. lemon zest, freshly squeezed (about 2 lemons)
- 1/4 cup fresh lemon juice, divided
- 4 oz. fish fillets (cod or salmon is best)
- 1/2 tsp. salt, divided
- 1/8 tsp. freshly ground black pepper, divided
- 4 green onions, thinly sliced (about 1/2 cup)

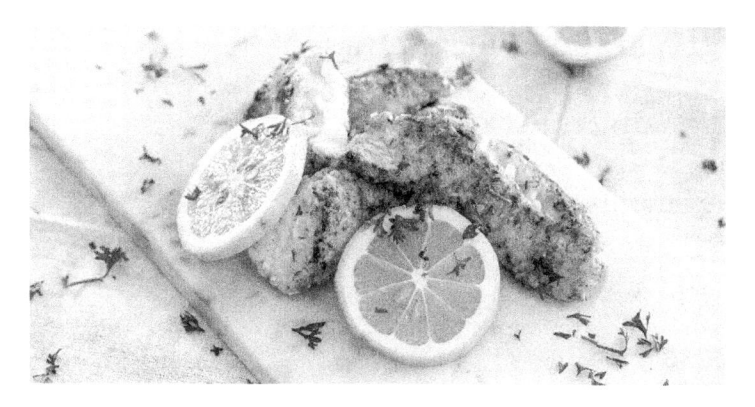

Directions:

1. Heat the oil in a large skillet over medium-high heat then add lemon zest and sauté for about 2 minutes. Add fish to the pan and season with salt, pepper, and lemon juice. Cover with a lid or aluminum foil. Cook for about four minutes or until the fish is white then turn off the heat. Add in green onions and serve immediately.

Nutrition:

- Calories: 125
- Fat: 6 g
- Carbohydrates: 3 g
- Fiber: 0.5 g
- Sugar: 1 g
- Protein: 13 g

31. Salmon Skewers in Cured Ham

Preparation time: 10 Mins

Cooking time: 15 Minutes

Servings: 4

Ingredients:

Salmon skewers:

- 60 ml finely chopped fresh basil
- 450 g salmon
- Salt and black pepper to taste
- 100 g dried ham sliced
- 1 tbsp. olive oil
- 8 pieces wooden skewers
- Water

Innings:

- 225 ml mayonnaise

Nutrition:

- Calories: 680
- Carbohydrates: 1 g
- Fats: 62 g
- Proteins: 28 g

Directions:

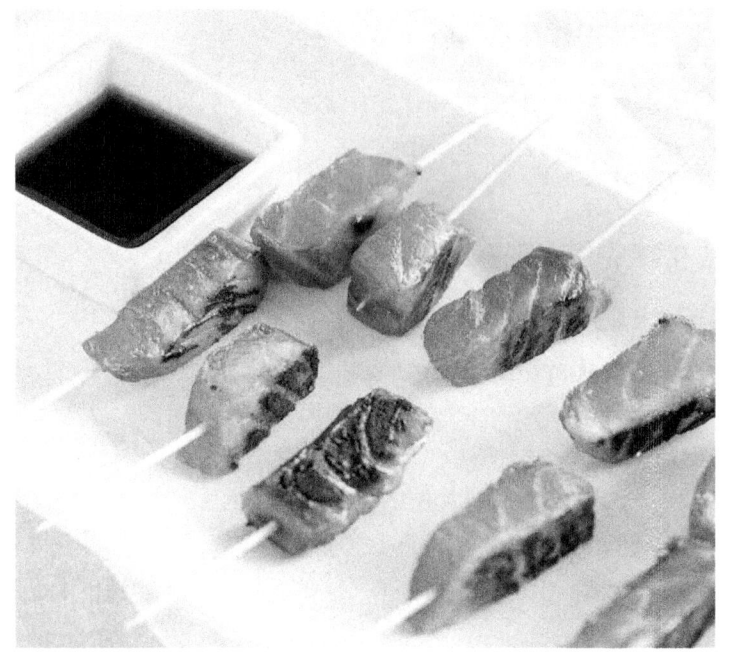

1. Soak the skewers in water.
2. Finely chop fresh basil.
3. Cut salmon fillet into rectangular pieces and fasten-on skewers.
4. Roll each kebab in the basil and pepper.
5. Cut the cured ham into thin slices and wrap her every kebab.
6. Sprinkle with olive oil and fry in a pan, grill, or in the oven.
7. Serve with mayonnaise or salad

32. Cod Loin with Horseradish and Browned Butter

Preparation time: 15 mins

Cooking time: 15 to 20 mins

Servings: 2

Ingredients:

- 1 1/2 lb. cod fillets, skinned
- 2 pinches ground black pepper, divided
- 2 pinches fresh grated nutmeg, divided
- 1/2 tsp. salt, divided
- 1/4 cup butter or ghee (1/4 stick), grated and at room temperature
- 4 oz. of your favorite horseradish sauce (about 1/3 cup)
- 2 tbsp. heavy cream or half-and-half (optional)

Nutrition:

- Calories: 295
- Fat: 16 g
- Carbohydrates: 4 g
- Fiber: 1 g
- Sugar: 0.5 g
- Protein: 31 g

Directions:

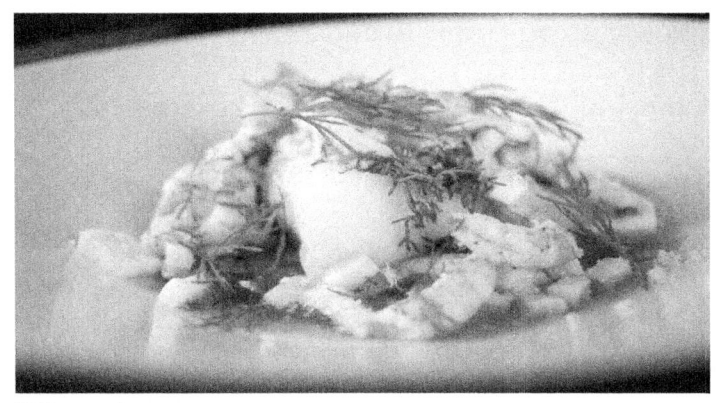

1. Heat oven to 375°F then arranges a baking sheet with parchment paper. Rinse the fish and pat dry with paper towels. Season with pepper and nutmeg; drizzle with butter, then season again with salt. Arrange a layer of fish on the baking sheet then sprinkle with one pinch of salt and one pinch of pepper. Continue until all fish is in the pan. Bake for about 15 to 20 minutes or until fish flakes when tested with a fork; set aside.
2. Heat oven to 450°F then adds the butter to a small skillet over medium heat. Cook butter until browned and bubbly. Add horseradish sauce then cream (if desired) to the pan; stir together until hot and well combined in an even sauce. Serve cod fillets with the sauce drizzled over top, garnished with additional nutmeg if desired.

33. Keto Seafood Chowder

Preparation time: 10 mins

Cooking time: 20-30 minutes

Servings: 2

Ingredients:

- 1 medium onion, diced
- 2 celery stalks, diced
- 2 tbsp. butter or ghee
- 1 cup heavy cream or half-and-half (optional)
- 1/2 cup clam juice (about 2 cans)
- 2 cups chicken stock or chicken broth (about 8 oz.)
- 4 oz. cooked shrimp (about 1 1/2 cups)
- Sea salt and freshly ground black pepper to taste
- 2 inches of water

Directions:

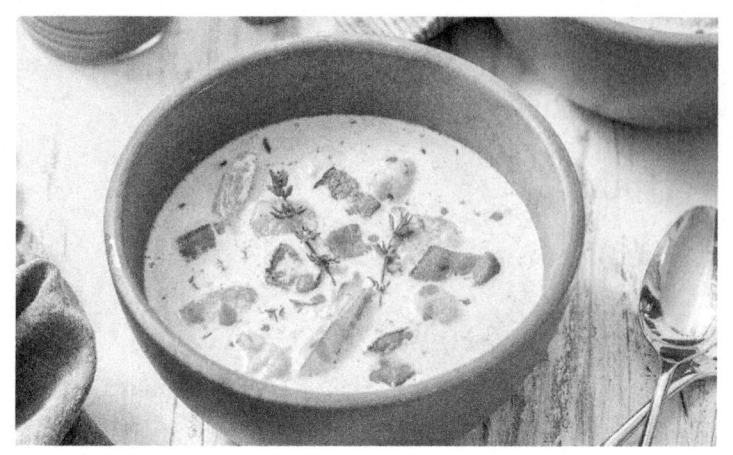

1. Heat a large pot with about 2 inches of water over medium heat then add onions and celery; cook for about five minutes until softened then add in the butter/ghee. Cook for another minute then pour in heavy cream/half-and-half and clam juice; bring to a boil. Add the broth and shrimp, then reduce heat to a simmer; cook for about 15 minutes or until seafood is cooked through. Season with salt and pepper as desired, then serve immediately.

Nutrition:

- Calories: 181
- Fat: 12 g
- Carbohydrates: 5 g
- Fiber: 0.5 g
- Sugar: 3 g
- Protein: 9 g

34. Creamy Keto Fish Casserole

Preparation time: 25 mins

Servings: 2

Ingredients:

- 4 tbsp. butter or ghee, melted
- 1/2 lb. tilapia fillet, thawed and cut into bite-size pieces
- 1 medium red bell pepper, chopped (optional)
- Sea salt and freshly ground black pepper to taste
- Parmesan cheese to taste
- Parsley to taste
- Lemon slices to taste

Nutrition:

- Calories: 296
- Fat: 18 g
- Carbohydrates: 2.6 g
- Fiber: 0 g
- Sugar: 0 g
- Protein: 26.4 g

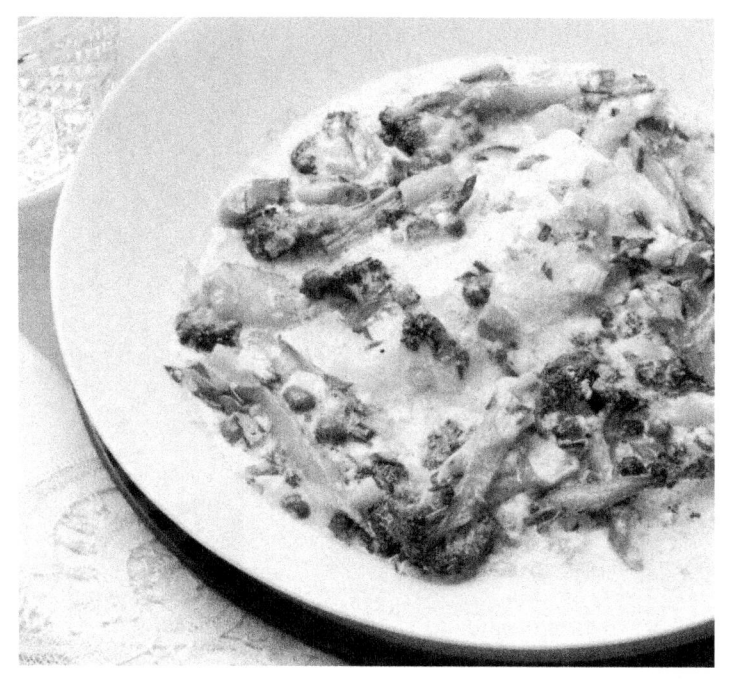

Directions:

1. Preheat oven to 350°F. Combine butter and seasonings in a small bowl; place on the fish pieces, coating thoroughly. Arrange fish in an 8x11 or 9x13 baking dish; bake for about 15 minutes until cooked through. Alternatively, you can broil for about 5 minutes or until lightly golden browned. Remove from heat and top with Parmesan cheese, parsley and lemon slices; serve immediately.

35. Coconut Mahi-Mahi Nuggets

Preparation time: 10 Mins

Cooking time: 10 Minutes

Servings: 2

Ingredients:

- 1 cup avocado oil or coconut oil, plus more as needed
- 1 lb. frozen mahi-mahi, thawed
- 2 large eggs
- 2 tbsp. avocado oil mayonnaise
- 1 cup almond flour
- 1/2 cup shredded coconut
- 1/4 cup crushed macadamia nuts
- Salt to taste
- Freshly ground black pepper to taste
- 1/2 lime, cut into wedges
- 1/4 cup dairy-free tartar sauce

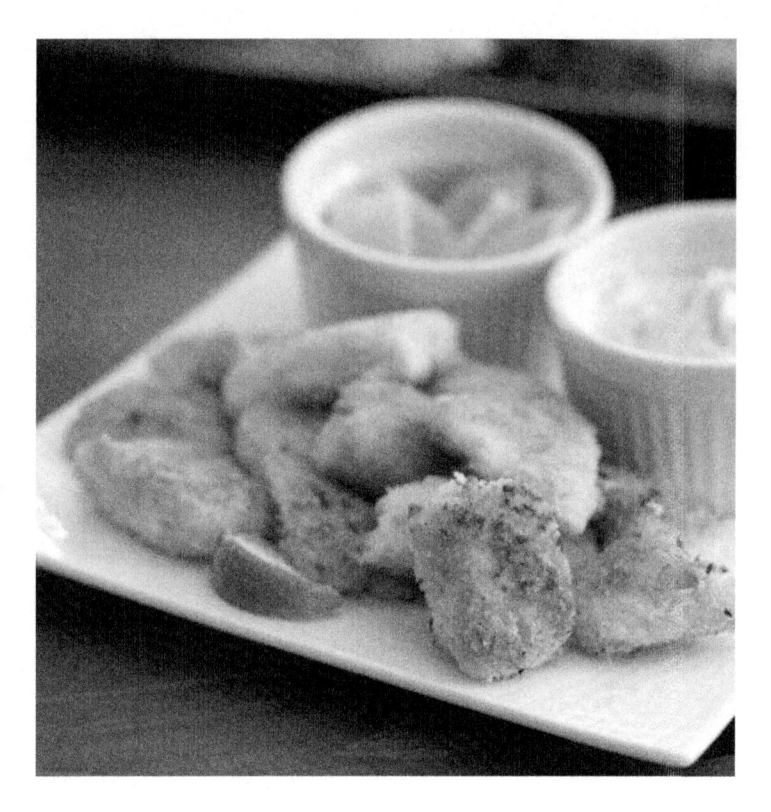

Directions:

1. In a skillet, warm the avocado oil at high heat. You want the oil to be about 1/2 inch deep, so adjust the amount of oil-based on the size of your pan.
2. Pat the fish to try using paper towels to take off any excess water.
3. In a small bowl, put and combine the eggs and mayonnaise.
4. In a medium mixing bowl, put and combine the almond flour, coconut, and macadamia

Nutrition:

- Calories: 733
- Fat: 53 g
- Carbohydrates: 10 g
- Fiber: 6 g
- Net Carbohydrates: 4 g
- Protein: 54 g

nuts. Season with salt and pepper. Cut the mahi-mahi into nuggets.

5. Put the fish into the egg mixture then dredge in the dry mix. Press into the dry mixture so that "breading" sticks well on all sides.
6. Add the fish into the hot oil. It should sizzle when you add the nuggets. Cook for 2 minutes per side, until golden and crispy.
7. Place the cooked nuggets on a paper towel-lined plate and squirt the lime wedges and tartar sauce over them.

veggies
&
dips

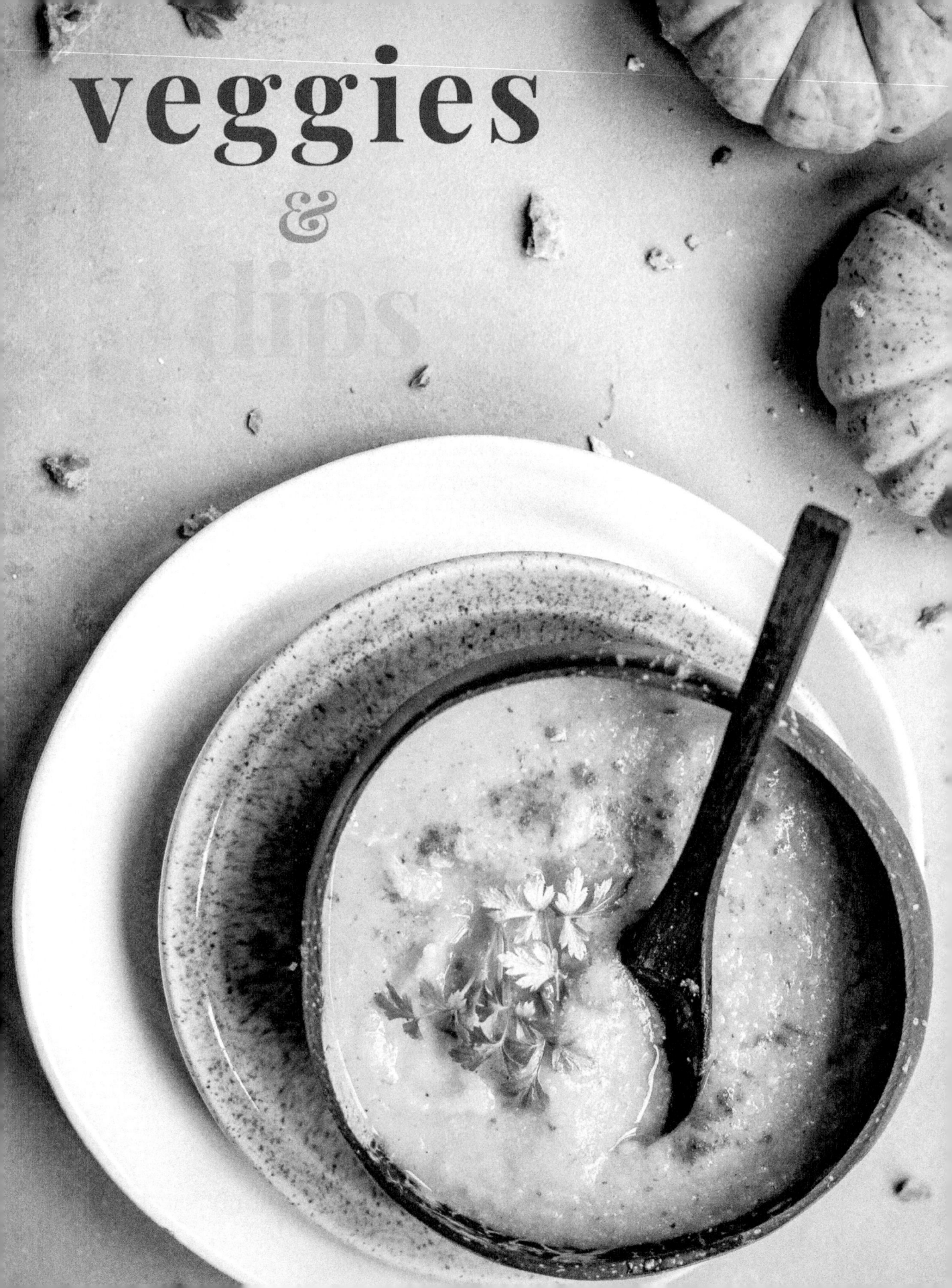

Vegetables and Dips

36. Radish, Carrot and Cilantro Salad

Preparation time: 15 mins

Cooking time: 0 minutes

Servings: 2

Ingredients:

- 1 1/2 lb. carrots
- 1/4 cup cilantro
- 1 1/2 lb. radish
- 1/2 tsp. salt
- 6 onions
- 1/4 tsp. black pepper
- 3 tbsp. lemon juice
- 3 tbsp. orange juice
- 2 tbsp. olive oil

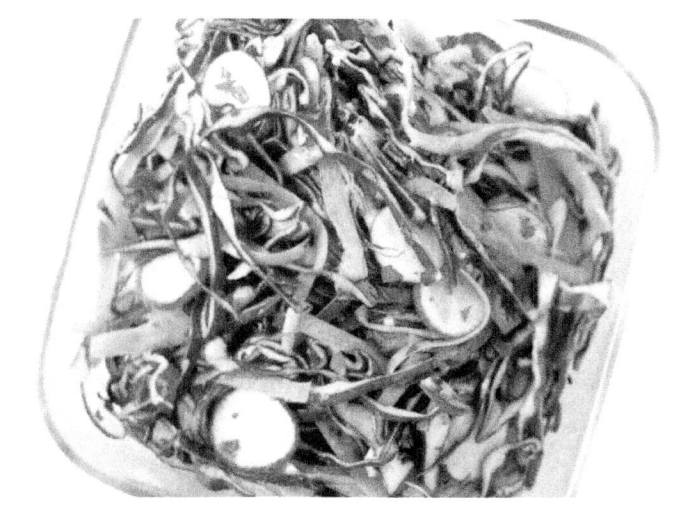

Directions:

1. Mix all the items until they merged properly.
2. Chill and serve.

Nutrition:

- Calories: 33
- Carbohydrates: 7 g
- Fat: 0 g
- Protein: 0 g

37. Lebanese Lemony Fattoush Fusion

Preparation time: 10 mins

Cooking time: 5 minutes

Servings: 2

Ingredients:

- 2 loaves whole-wheat pita bread
- 3 tbsp. extra-virgin olive oil
- Salt and pepper to taste
- 1/2 tsp. sumac
- 5 pieces Roma tomatoes, chopped
- 5 pieces radishes stem removed, thinly sliced
- 5 pieces green onions, chopped
- 2 cups fresh parsley leaves stem removed, chopped
- 1-piece English cucumber, chopped
- 1 heart Romaine lettuce, chopped

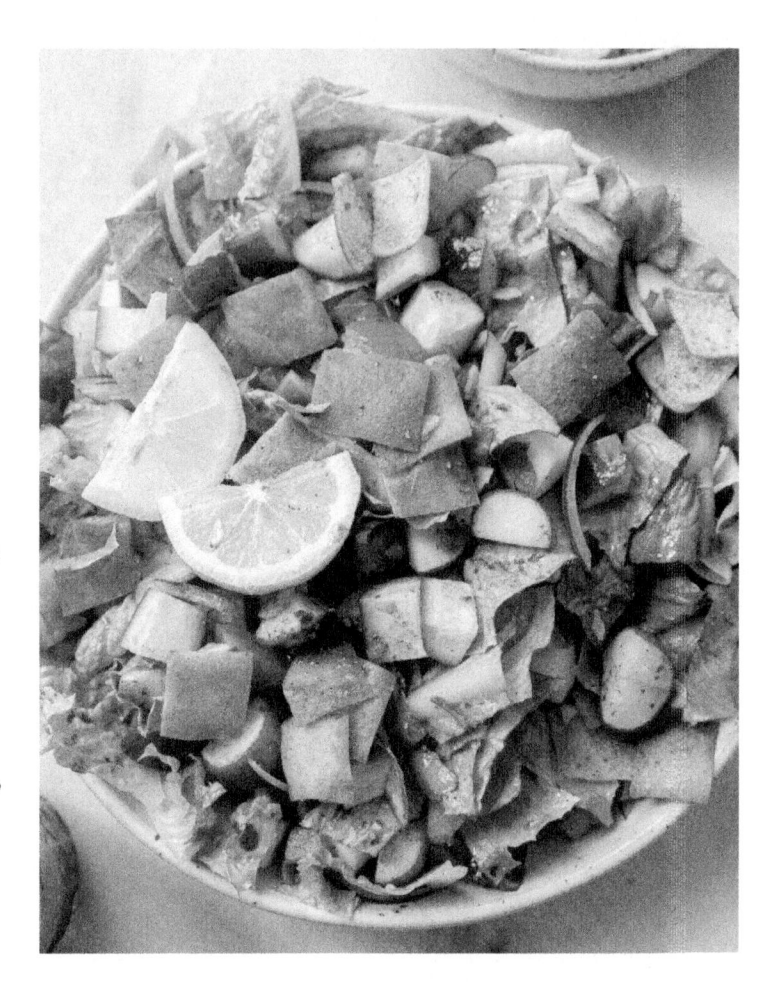

Directions:

1. In your toaster oven, toast the pita bread for 2 minutes until turning crisp, but is not browned.
2. Heat 3 tbsp. olive oil in a large frying pan. Cut the toasted pita bread into pieces and add them to the pan. Fry the broken pita pieces for 3 minutes until browned, tossing

- 1 cup fresh mint leaves, chopped (optional)

Dressing:

- Salt and pepper to taste
- 1 tsp. ground sumac or lemon zest
- 1 1/2 lime juice
- 1/3 cup extra-virgin olive oil
- 1/4 tsp. ground cinnamon
- 1/4 tsp. ground allspice

Nutrition:

- Calories: 478.8
- Fat: 18.1 g
- Fiber: 3.7 g
- Carbohydrates: 32.1 g
- Protein: 21.3 g

frequently. Season the pita chips with salt, pepper, and sumac. Remove the seasoned pita chips from the heat and place them on paper towels to drain.

3. Combine the remainder of the salad ingredients in a large mixing bowl. Mix until fully combined.
4. Combine and whisk together all the dressing ingredients in a separate smaller mixing bowl. Mix well until fully combined.
5. Drizzle the lime-vinaigrette dressing over the salad. Toss gently to coat evenly.
6. Add the oil-drained pita chips and toss gently again until fully combined.

38. Cucumber Yogurt Salad

Preparation time: 10 minutes

Cooking time: 0 minutes

Servings: 2

Ingredients:

- 2 peeled and diced English cucumbers
- 1 1/2 tbsp. fresh garlic, crushed
- A pinch of salt
- 2 tsp. dried mint
- 1/8 tbsp. fresh dill, already minced
- 1-quart low-fat yogurt, plain

Directions:

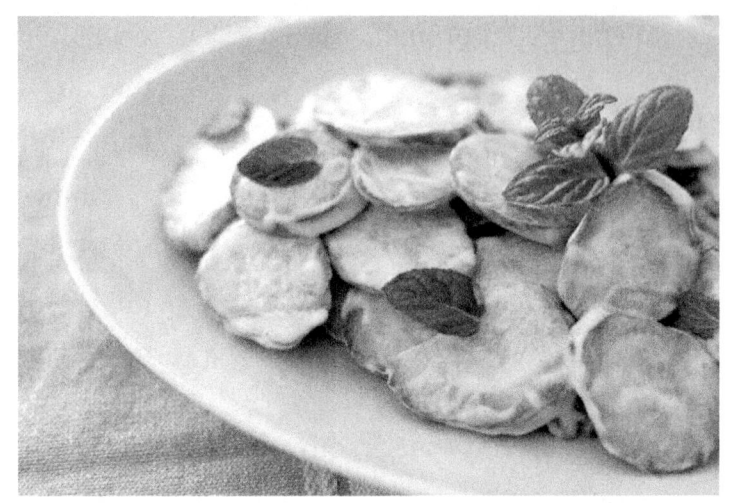

1. In a small bowl, mix the dill, garlic, and salt.
2. Pour the yogurt in and mix well.
3. Add cucumber, mint and stir well
4. Put inside the refrigerator to chill, then serve.

Nutrition:

- Calories: 167
- Carbohydrates: 21 g
- Fat: 4 g
- Protein: 13 g

39. White Beans with Vegetables

Preparation time: 10 mins

Cooking time: 0 mins

Servings: 2

Ingredients:

- 1/2 lb. white beans, cooked
- 1 onion, chopped
- 1 tbsp. lemon juice
- 7–8 cherry tomatoes, chopped
- 1 tbsp. oregano
- Ground pepper, to taste
- 2–3 tbsp. cilantro, chopped
- Salt, to taste

Nutrition:

- Calories: 345
- Fat: 27 g
- Carbohydrates: 67 g
- Protein: 21 g

Directions:

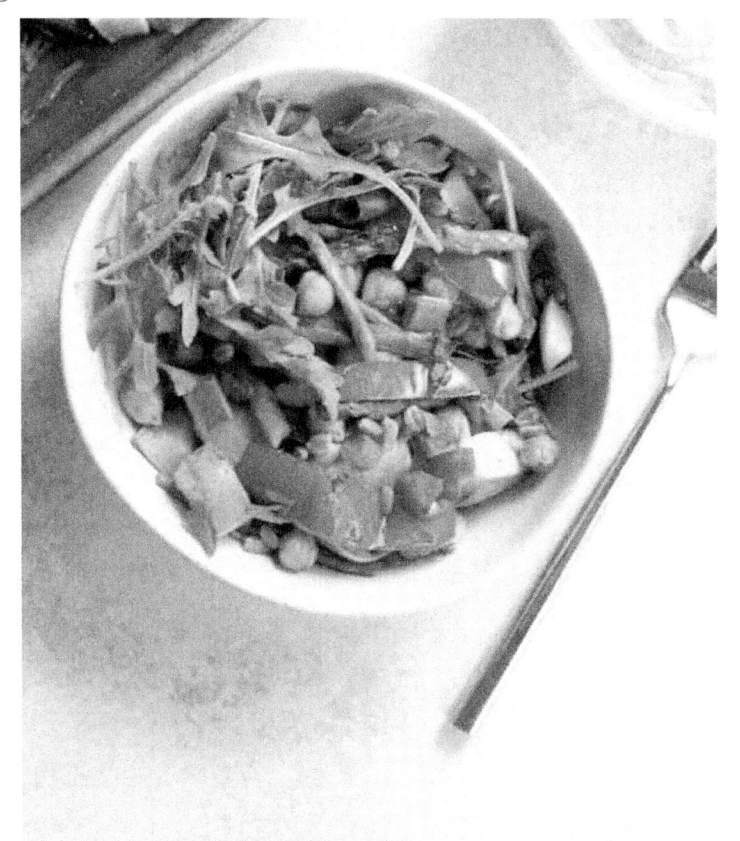

1. In a large bowl combine white beans, onion, tomatoes, cilantro, oregano, salt, pepper, and lemon juice.
2. Add mixture to a serving dish.
3. Enjoy.

40. Garlicky Sautéed Zucchini with Mint

Preparation time: 5 Minutes

Cooking time: 10 Minutes

Servings: 4

Ingredients:

- 3 large green zucchinis
- 3 tbsp. extra-virgin olive oil
- 1 large onion, chopped
- 3 garlic cloves, minced
- 1 tsp. dried mint
- Salt to taste

Nutrition:

- Calories: 147
- Carbohydrates: 12 g
- Protein: 4 g

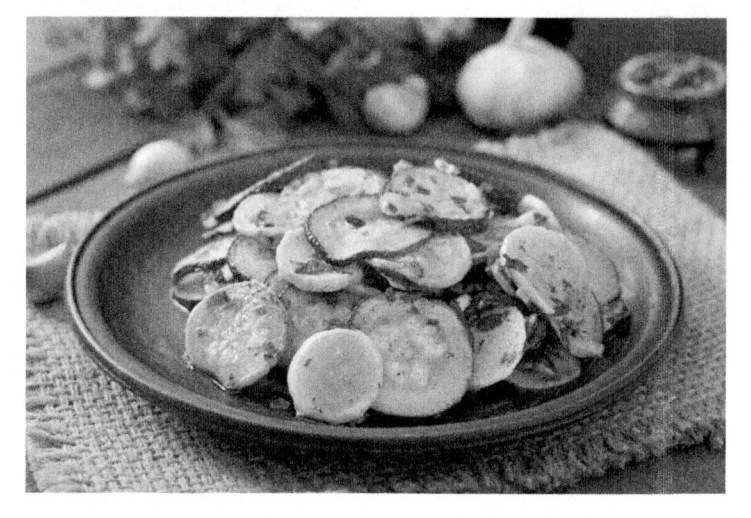

Directions:

1. Cut the zucchini into 1/2-inch cubes.
2. Using a huge skillet, place over medium heat, cook the olive oil, onions, and garlic for 3 minutes, stirring constantly.
3. Add the zucchini and salt to the skillet and toss to combine with the onions and garlic, cooking for 5 minutes.
4. Add the mint to the skillet, tossing to combine. Cook for another 2 minutes. Serve warm

41. Sautéed Garlic Spinach

Preparation time: 5 Minutes

Cooking time: 10 Minutes

Servings: 4

Ingredients:

- 1/4 cup extra-virgin olive oil
- 1 large onion, thinly sliced
- 3 garlic cloves, minced
- 6 (1 lb.) bags of baby spinach, washed
- 1 lemon, cut into wedges
- 1/2 tsp. salt.

Nutrition:

- Calories: 301
- Carbohydrates: 29 g
- Protein: 17 g

Directions:

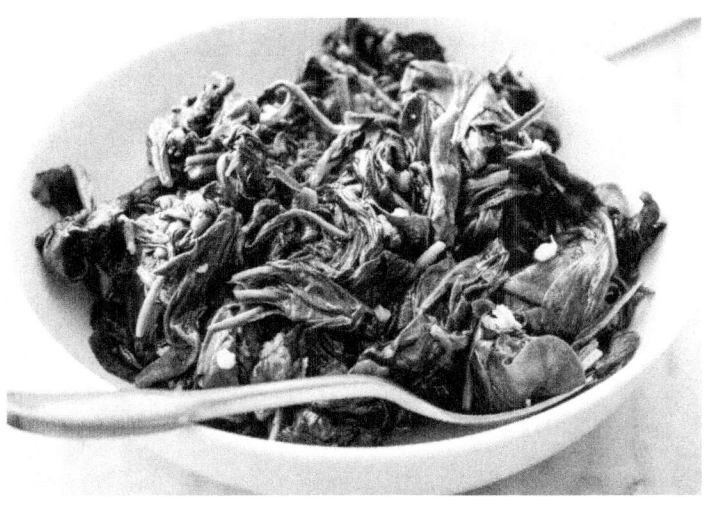

1. Cook the olive oil, onion, and garlic in a large skillet for 2 minutes over medium heat.
2. Add one bag of spinach and 1/2 tsp. salt. Cover the skillet and let the spinach wilt for 30 seconds. Repeat (omitting the salt), adding 1 bag of spinach at a time.
3. Once all the spinach has been added, remove the cover and cook for 3 minutes, letting some of the moisture evaporate.
4. Serve warm with lemon juice over the top.

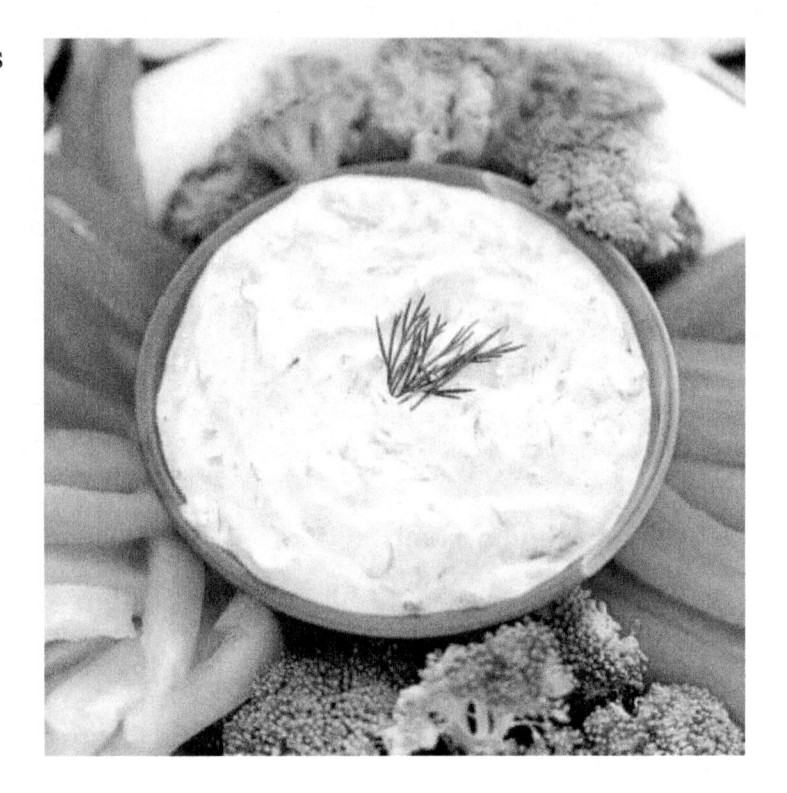

42. Easy Dill Dip

Preparation time: 5 minutes

Servings: 2

Ingredients:

- 1 cup sour cream (not plain)
- 2 tsp. dill pickle relish (not sweetened)
- 2 tbsp. white wine vinegar (not balsamic)
- 1 tsp. celery seed (to mellow the flavor, can substitute with garlic powder)

Nutrition:

- Calories: 43
- Fat: 4 g
- Carbohydrates: 0.9 g
- Fiber: 0.1 g
- Sugar: 0.5 g
- Protein: 1.2 g

Directions:

1. Place all ingredients in a small mixing bowl; whisk to combine. Chill for at least 30 minutes before serving. This dip tastes best when served within a few hours of its preparation so it is best to make a big batch and store it in the refrigerator until ready to serve.

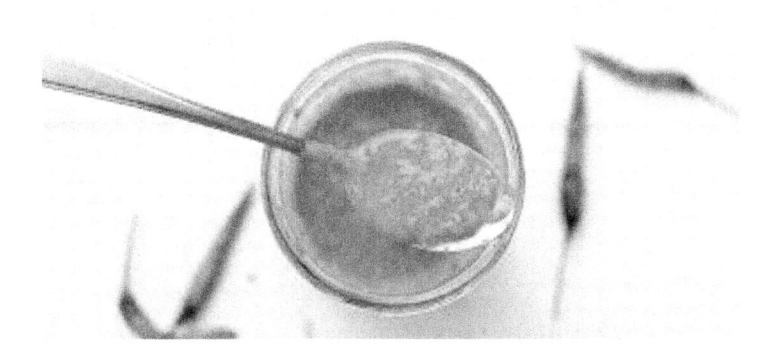

43. Peri-Peri Sauce

Preparation time: 10 Mins

Cooking time: 5 Minutes

Servings: 4

Ingredients:

- 1 tomato, chopped
- 1 red onion, chopped
- 1 red bell pepper, deseeded and chopped
- 1 red chili, deseeded and chopped
- 4 garlic cloves, minced
- 2 tbsp. extra-virgin olive oil
- Juice of 1 lemon
- 1 tbsp. dried oregano
- 1 tbsp. smoked paprika
- 1 tsp. sea salt

Nutrition:

- Calories: 98
- Fat: 6.5 g
- Carbohydrates: 7.8 g
- Fiber: 3.0 g
- Sodium: 295 mg
- Protein: 1.0 g

Directions:

1. Process all the fixings in a food processor or a blender until smooth.
2. Transfer the mixture to a small saucepan over medium-high heat and bring to a boil, stirring often.
3. Reduce the heat to medium and allow to simmer for 5 minutes until heated through.
4. You can store the sauce in an airtight container in the refrigerator for up to 5 days.

44. Spicy Mediterranean Feta Dip

Preparation time: 10 mins

Servings: 2

Ingredients:

- 4 oz. Feta
- 1 cup plain Greek yogurt (not Greek style)
- 1 tbsp. fresh lemon juice (about 1 lemon)
- 2 garlic cloves, minced
- 1 jalapeño pepper, seeded and finely chopped (about 1 tsp.)
- 1/4 tsp. salt

Nutrition:

- Calories: 116
- Fat: 8 g
- Carbohydrates: 2 g
- Fiber: 0 g
- Sugar: 1 g
- Protein: 9.5 g

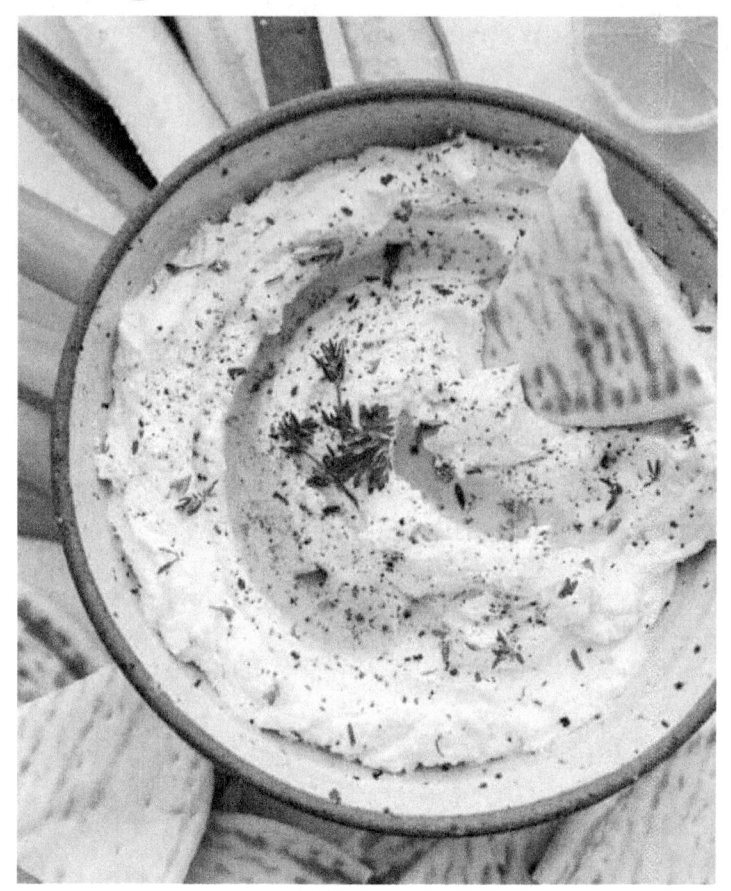

Directions:

1. In a medium bowl, combine all ingredients. Cover and refrigerate for at least 30 minutes before serving. Best when served within several hours of preparation. Serve with pita wedges, crackers, or vegetables of choice.

45. Radishes and Ranch Dirt Dip

Preparation time: 5 minutes

Servings: 2

Ingredients:

- 1 lb. radishes (about 1 1/2 cups), trimmed and very thinly sliced (about 3 cups)
- 2 garlic cloves, minced
- 1/4 cup sour cream or Greek yogurt (not plain)
- 1/4 cup mayonnaise or salad dressing (not salad dressing)
- 1/8 tsp. salt
- 1/2 cup shredded cheddar cheese (about 2 oz.)

Nutrition:

- Calories: 83
- Fat: 4 g
- Carbohydrates: 2 g
- Fiber: 0.1 g
- Sugar: 0 g
- Protein: 3.2 g

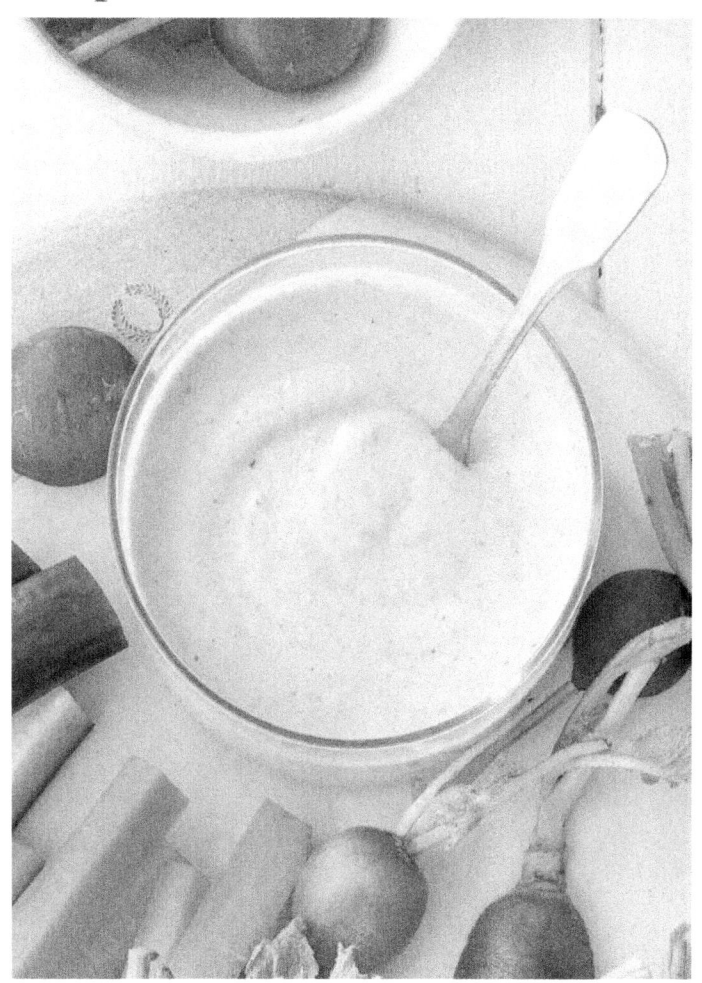

Directions:

1. In a medium mixing bowl, combine radishes, garlic, sour cream, mayonnaise, salt, and cheddar cheese mix well. Serve immediately with pita wedges or crackers.

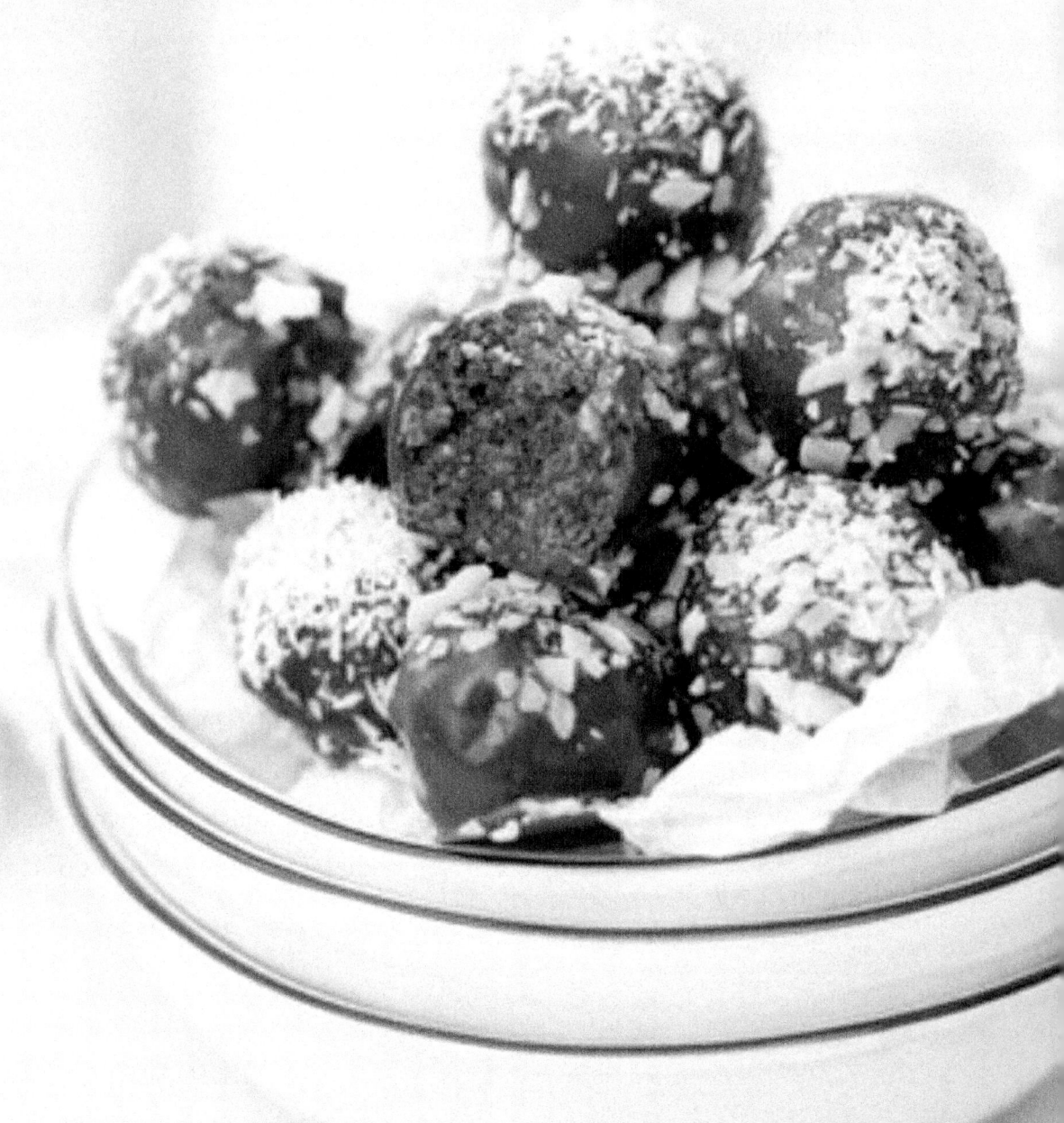

sweets & fruits

Sweets and Fruit

46. Delicious Coffee Ice Cream

Preparation time: 10 mins

Cooking time: 5 minutes

Servings: 1

Ingredients:

- 6 oz. coconut cream, frozen into ice cubes
- 1 ripe avocado, diced and frozen
- 1/2 cup coffee Expresso
- 2 tbsp. sweetener
- 1 tsp. vanilla extract
- 1 tbsp. water
- Coffee beans to taste

Nutrition:

- Calories: 596
- Carbohydrates: 20.5 g
- Fat: 61 g
- Protein: 6.3 g

Directions:

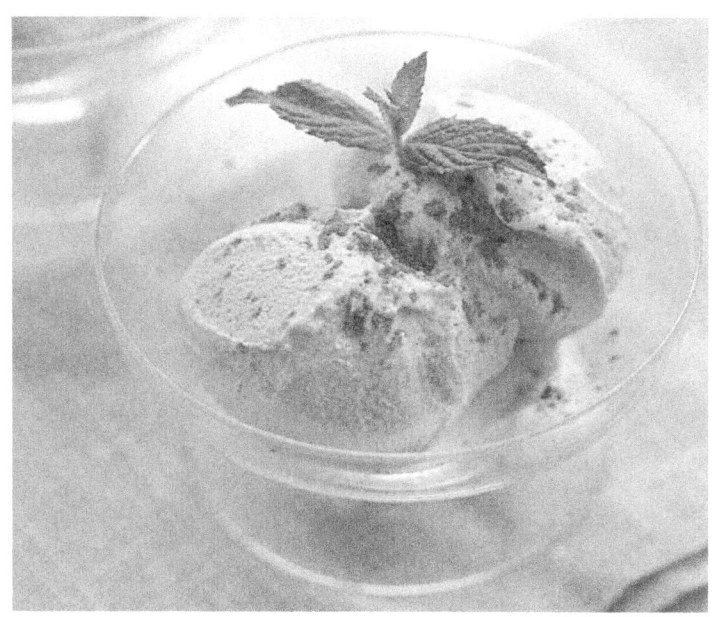

1. Take out the frozen coconut cubes and avocado from the fridge. Slightly melt them for 5 to 10 minutes.
2. Add the sweetener, coffee expresso, and vanilla extract to the coconut avocado mix and whisk with an immersion blender until it becomes creamy (for about 1 minute). Pour in the water and blend for 30 seconds.
3. Top with coffee beans and enjoy!

47. Chocolate Spread with Hazelnuts

Preparation time: 5 minutes

Cooking time: 5 minutes

Servings: 6

Ingredients:

- 2 tbsp. cacao powder
- 5 oz. hazelnuts, roasted and without shells
- 1 oz. unsalted butter
- 1/4 cup of coconut oil

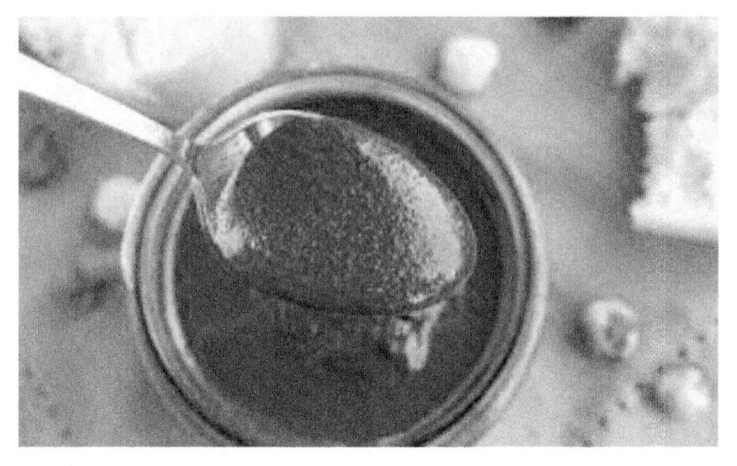

Directions:

1. Whisk all the spread ingredients with a blender.
2. Serve.

Nutrition:

- Calories: 271
- Carbohydrates: 2 g
- Fat: 28 g
- Protein: 4 g

48. Chocolate Mug Muffins

Preparation time: 5 minutes

Cooking time: 2 minutes

Servings: 4

Ingredients:

- 4 tbsp. almond flour
- 1 tsp. baking powder
- 4 tbsp. granulated erythritol
- 2 tbsp. cocoa powder
- 1/2 tsp. vanilla extract
- 2 pinches of salt
- 2 eggs beaten
- 3 tbsp. butter, melted
- 1 tsp. coconut oil, for greasing the mug
- 1/2 oz. sugar-free dark chocolate, chopped

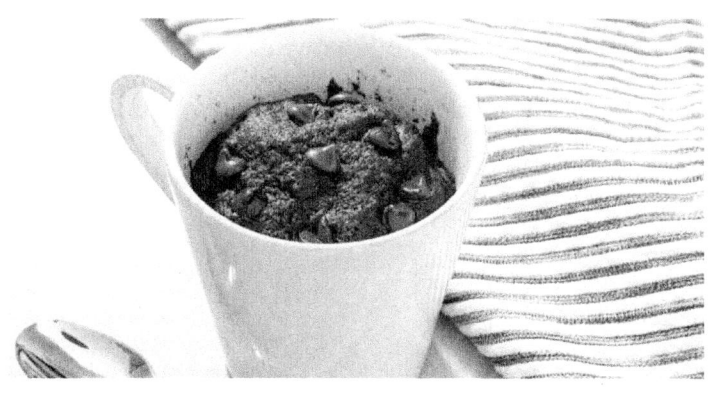

Directions:

1. Mix the dry ingredients in a separate bowl. Add the melted butter, beaten eggs, and chocolate to the bowl. Stir thoroughly.
2. Divide your dough into four pieces. Put these pieces in the greased mugs and put them in the microwave. Cook for 1–1 1/2 minutes (700 watts).
3. Let them cool for 1 minute and serve.

Nutrition:

- Calories: 208
- Carbohydrates: 2 g
- Fat: 19 g
- Protein: 5 g

49. Keto and Dairy-Free Vanilla Custard

Preparation time: 11 minutes

Cooking time: 5 minutes

Servings: 4

Ingredients:

- 6 egg yolks
- 1/2 cup unsweetened almond milk
- 1 tsp. vanilla extract
- 1/4 cup melted coconut oil
- Water

Nutrition:

- Calories: 215.38
- Carbohydrates: 1 g
- Fat: 21 g
- Protein: 4 g

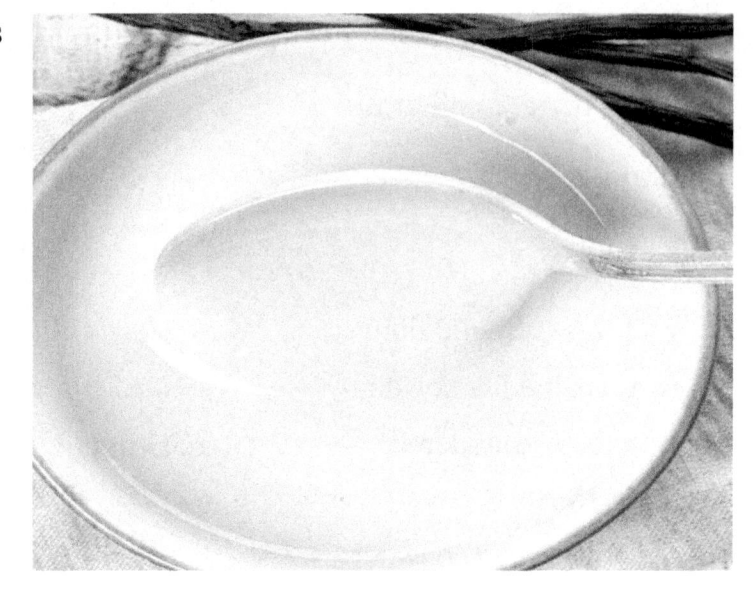

Directions:

1. Mix egg yolks, almond milk, and vanilla in a metal bowl.
2. Gradually stir in the melted coconut oil.
3. Boil water in a saucepan, place the mixing bowl over the saucepan.
4. Whisk the mixture constantly and vigorously until thickened for about 5 minutes.
5. Remover from the saucepan, serve hot or chill in the fridge.

50. Matcha Skillet Soufflé

Preparation time: 5 minutes

Cooking time: 5 minutes

Servings: 1

Ingredients:

- 3 large eggs
- 2 tbsp. sweetener
- 1 tsp. vanilla extract
- 1 tbsp. matcha powder
- 1 tbsp. butter
- 7 whole raspberries
- 1 tbsp. coconut oil
- 1 tbsp. unsweetened cocoa powder
- 1/4 cup whipped cream

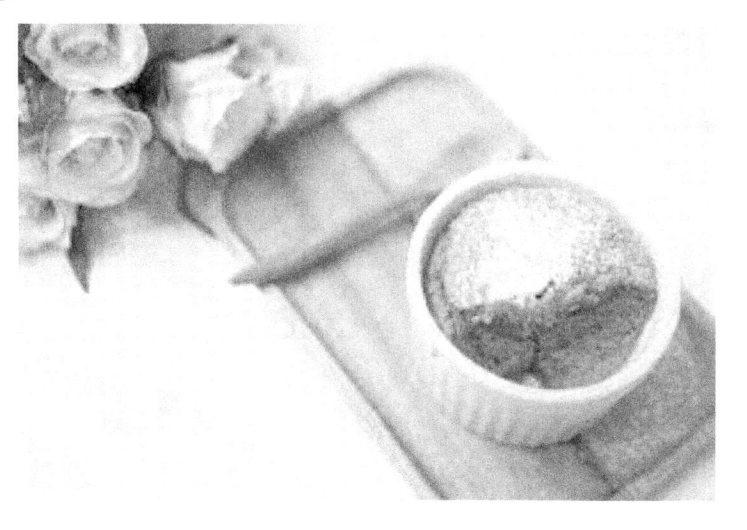

Directions:

1. Broil, then heat up a heavy-bottom pan over medium heat.
2. Whip the egg whites with 1 tablespoon of Swerve confectioners. Once the peaks form to add in the matcha powder, whisk again.
3. With a fork, break up the yolks. Mix in the vanilla, then adds a little amount of the whipped whites. Carefully fold the remaining whites into the yolk mixture.
4. Dissolve the butter in a pan, put the soufflé mixture in the pan. Reduce the heat to low and top with raspberries. Cook until the eggs double in size and set.

Nutrition:

- Calories: 578
- Fat: 50.91 g
- Carbohydrates: 5.06 g
- Protein: 20.95 g

5. Transfer the pan to the oven and keep an eye on it. Cook until golden browned.
6. Melt the coconut oil and combine with cocoa powder, whipped cream, and the remaining Swerve.
7. Drizzle the chocolate mixture across the top.

51. Oat and Fruit Parfait

Preparation time: 5 minutes

Cooking time: 10 minutes

Servings: 2

Ingredients:

- 1/2 cup whole-grain rolled or quick-cooking oats (not instant)
- 1/2 cup walnut pieces
- 1 tsp. honey
- 1 cup sliced fresh strawberries
- 1 1/2 cups (12 oz.) vanilla low-fat Greek yogurt
- Fresh mint leaves for garnish

Nutrition:

- Calories: 385
- Fat: 17 g
- Carbohydrates: 35 g
- Protein: 21 g

Directions:

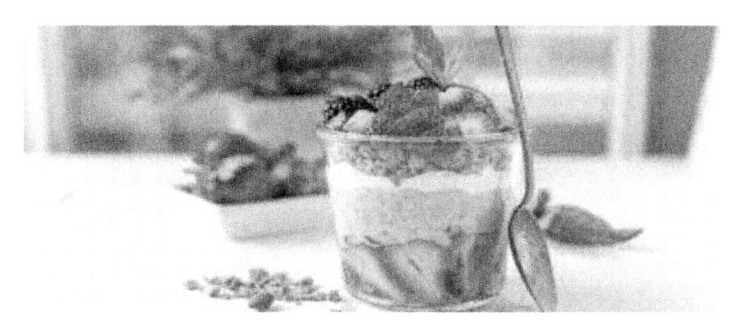

1. Preheat the oven to 300°F.
2. Spread the oats and walnuts in a single layer on a baking sheet
3. Toast the oats and nuts just until you begin to smell the nuts, 10 to 12 minutes. Remove the pan from the oven and set it aside.
4. In a small microwave-safe bowl, heat the honey just until warm, about 30 seconds. Add the strawberries and stir to coat.
5. Place 1 tablespoon of the strawberries in the bottom of each of 2 dessert dishes or 8 oz. glasses.
6. Add a portion of yogurt and then a portion of oats and repeat the layers until the containers are full, ending with the berries and mint leaves. Serve immediately or chill until ready to eat.

52. Deliciously Cold Lychee Sorbet

Preparation time: 10 mins

Cooking time: 5 minutes

Servings: 2

Ingredients:

- 2 cups fresh lychees, pitted and sliced
- 2 tbsp. honey
- Mint leaves for garnish

Nutrition:

- Calories: 151
- Carbohydrates: 38.9 g
- Fat: 0.4 g
- Protein: 0.7 g

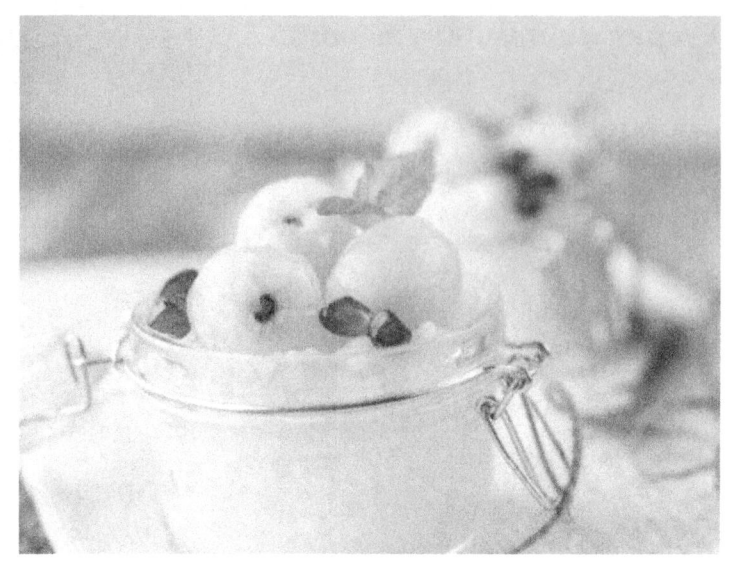

Directions:

1. Place the lychee slices and honey in a food processor
2. Pulse until smooth.
3. Pour in a container and place inside the fridge for at least two hours.
4. Scoop the sorbet and serve with mint leaves.

53. Creamed Fruit Salad

Preparation time: 10 mins

Cooking time: 0 mins

Servings: 2

Ingredients:

- 1 orange, peeled and sliced
- 2 apples, pitted and diced
- 2 peaches, pitted and diced
- 1 cup seedless grapes
- 3/4 cup Greek-style yogurt, well-chilled
- 3 tbsp. honey

Nutrition:

- Calories: 250
- Fat: 0.7 g
- Carbohydrates: 60 g
- Protein: 6.4 g

Directions:

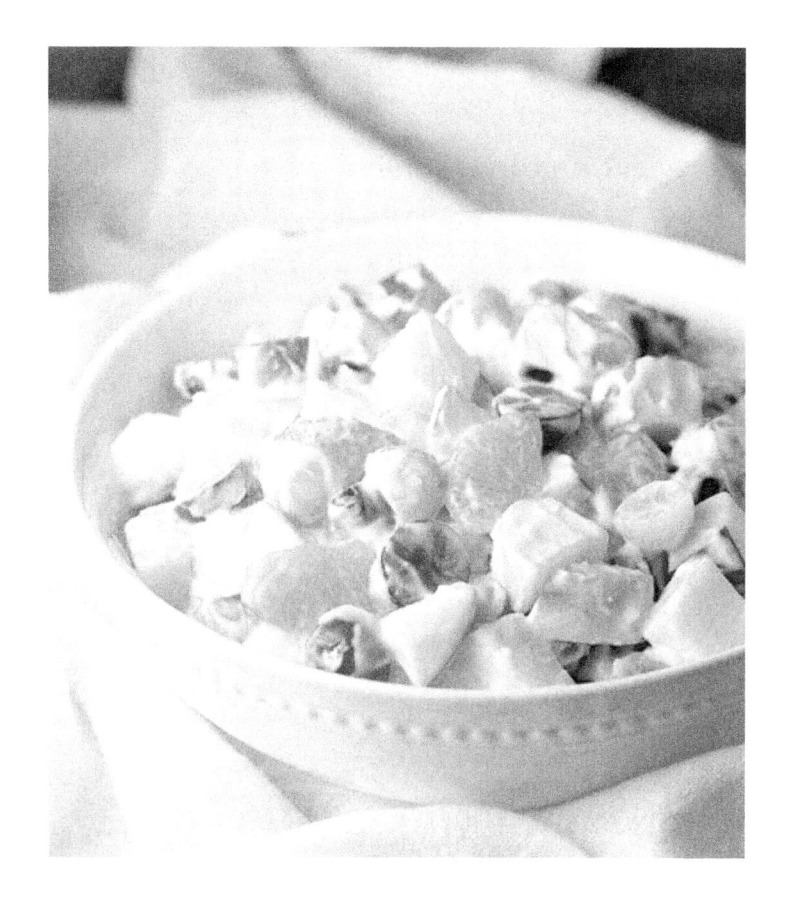

1. Divide the fruits between dessert bowls.
2. Top with the yogurt. Add a few drizzles of honey to each serving and serve well-chilled.
3. Bon appétit!

54. Strawberry, Blueberry, Lemon Juice, Ginger and Brown Sugar Salad

Preparation time: 10 mins

Cooking time: 15 minutes

Servings: 2

Ingredients:

- 1 lb. strawberries (about 4–5 medium), washed and dried
- 2 scoops of whey protein powder (about 10 oz.)
- 2 cups water plus ice cubes (or almond milk)
- 1/4 cup coconut oil, melted (plus more for greasing the bowl)
- 1 cup fresh blueberries or frozen blueberries, thawed (about 2 oz.) or about 1 cup frozen blueberries (thawed as needed)
- 1/2 tsp. vanilla extract (optional)

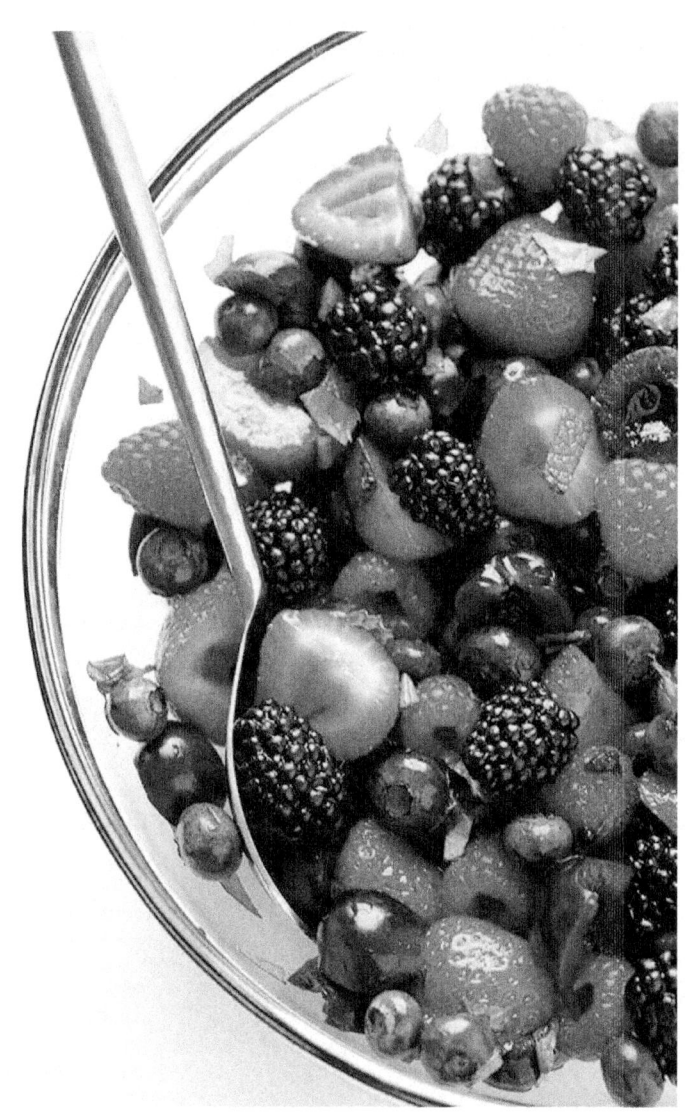

Directions:

1. Place berries on a large serving dish. Pour melted coconut oil over the berries and

- 1 cup Brown sugar
- 1 tbsp. Ginger
- 2 tbsp. Lemon juice

Nutrition:

- Calories: 162
- Fat: 14 g
- Carbohydrates: 2.9 g
- Fiber: 0.2 g
- Sugar: 1 g
- Protein: 9.2 g

drizzle with sugar-free syrup (if using) then sprinkle with protein powder.

2. Place four bowls over medium heat then add water, ice cubes (or almond milk), and whey protein powder to each bowl. Whisk frequently until the whey protein smooths out and is dissolved in the water/ice cubes. Add more ice cubes to each bowl as needed; bring to a simmer, stirring constantly until smooth and creamy (about 15 minutes).
3. Meanwhile, add brown sugar, ginger, lemon juice, vanilla extract, and blueberries into the blender; blend on a high setting until smooth (about 30 seconds). Pour into small glasses and serve immediately.

55. Greek Frozen Yogurt Dessert

Preparation time: 10 minutes

Cooking time: 0 minutes

Servings: 2

Ingredients:

- 1/2 pineapple, diced
- 2 cups Greek-style yogurt, frozen
- 3 oz. almonds, slivered

Nutrition:

- Calories: 307
- Fat: 14.4 g
- Carbohydrates: 29.1 g
- Protein: 18 g

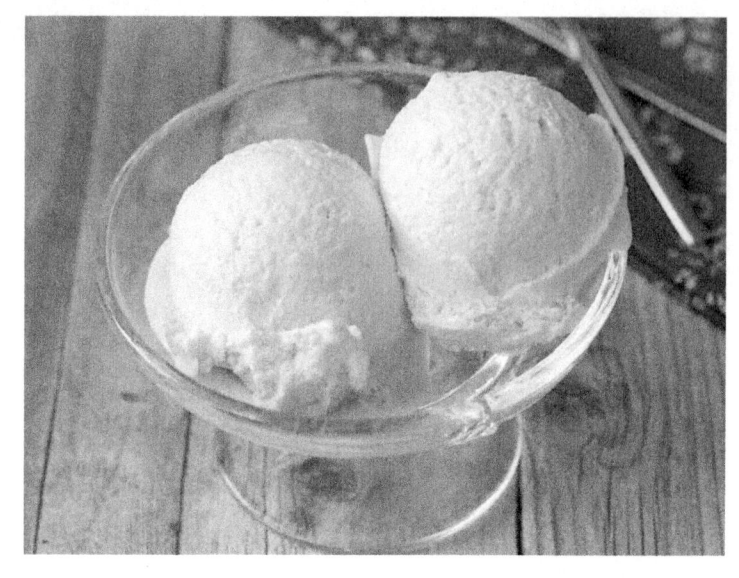

Directions:

1. Divide the pineapple between two dessert bowls. Spoon the yogurt over it.
2. Top with the slivered almonds.
3. Cover and place in your refrigerator until you're ready to serve. Bon appétit!

7. Measurement Conversion

Volume Equivalents (Liquid)

Type	US Standard (oz.)	Metric
2 tbsp.	1 fl. oz.	30 mL
1/4 cup	2 fl. oz.	60 mL
1/2 cup	4 fl. oz.	120 mL
1 cup	8 fl. oz.	240 mL

Volume Equivalents (Dry)

Type	Metric
1/4 tsp.	1 mL
1/2 tsp.	2 mL
1 tsp.	5 mL
1 tbsp.	15 mL
1/4 cup	59 mL
1/2 cup	118 mL
1 cup	235 mL

Oven Temperatures

Fahrenheit (°F)	Celsius (°C)
250	120
300	150
325	165
350	180
375	190
400	200
425	220
450	230

MEAL	MONDAY
BREAKFAST	
SNACK	
LUNCH	

8. 28 Days Eating Plan

Day	Breakfast	Lunch	Dinner	Desserts
1	Bacon and Avocado Omelet	Cilantro Chicken Breasts with Mayo-Avocado Sauce	Lamb Burgers with Tzatziki	Delicious Coffee Ice Cream
2	Keto Smoked Salmon with Avocado Slice	Sweet Garlic Chicken Skewers	Blackened Fish Tacos with Slaw	Chocolate Spread with Hazelnuts
3	Keto Cereal with Almond Milk and Walnuts	Lamb Burgers with Tzatziki	Thai Keto Tuna Salad Wrap	Chocolate Mug Muffins
4	Kale Fritters	Thai Keto Tuna Salad Wrap	Creamy Keto Fish Casserole	Keto and Dairy-Free Vanilla Custard
5	Cream Cheese Eggs	Keto Chinese Pork Stew with Cabbage	Coconut Mahi-Mahi Nuggets	Matcha Skillet Soufflé
6	Creamy Basil Baked Sausage	Lamb Sliders	Zingy Lemon Fish	Oat and Fruit Parfait
7	Strawberry Rhubarb Smoothie	Keto Zucchini Lasagna	Keto Seafood Chowder	Deliciously Cold Lychee Sorbet
8	Ricotta Cloud Pancakes	Blackened Fish Tacos with Slaw	Cilantro Chicken Breasts with Mayo-Avocado Sauce	Creamed Fruit Salad
9	Keto Cinnamon Coffee	Chicken Bacon Burger	Lamb Sliders	Strawberry, Blueberry, Lemon Juice, Ginger and Brown Sugar Salad
10	Keto Coconut Flake Balls	Zingy Lemon Fish	Keto Zucchini Lasagna	Greek Frozen Yogurt Dessert

11	Berry Smoothie	Garlic Steak Bite Salad with Tarragon Dressing	Salmon Skewers in Cured Ham	Delicious Coffee Ice Cream
12	Chocolate Banana Smoothie	Keto Pulled Pork with Roasted Tomato Salad	Cod Loin with Horseradish and Browned Butter	Chocolate Spread with Hazelnuts
13	Smoked Salmon and Poached Eggs on Toast	Lamb Burgers with Tzatziki	Garlic Steak Bite Salad with Tarragon Dressing	Chocolate Mug Muffins
14	Fruit Smoothie	Keto Harvest Pumpkin and Sausage Soup	Zingy Lemon Fish	Keto and Dairy-Free Vanilla Custard
15	Almond Coconut Egg Wraps	Salmon Skewers in Cured Ham	Chicken Bacon Burger	Matcha Skillet Soufflé
16	Bacon and Avocado Omelet	Keto Zucchini Lasagna	Lamb Sliders	Oat and Fruit Parfait
17	Keto Smoked Salmon with Avocado Slice	Creamy Keto Fish Casserole	Herby Fishcakes with Zucchini Salad	Deliciously Cold Lychee Sorbet
18	Keto Cereal with Almond Milk and Walnuts	Keto Seafood Chowder	Keto Pulled Pork with Roasted Tomato Salad	Creamed Fruit Salad
19	Kale Fritters	Herby Fishcakes with Zucchini Salad	Coconut Mahi-Mahi Nuggets	Strawberry, Blueberry, Lemon Juice, Ginger and Brown Sugar Salad
20	Cream Cheese Eggs	Stuffed Keto Mushrooms	Keto Chinese Pork Stew with Cabbage	Greek Frozen Yogurt Dessert

21	Creamy Basil Baked Sausage	Cilantro Chicken Breasts with Mayo-Avocado Sauce	Lamb Burgers with Tzatziki	Keto Coconut Flake Balls
22	Almond Coconut Egg Wraps	Sweet Garlic Chicken Skewers	Cod Loin with Horseradish and Browned Butter	Strawberry, Blueberry, Lemon Juice, Ginger and Brown Sugar Salad
23	Ricotta Cloud Pancakes	Coconut Mahi-Mahi Nuggets	Keto Harvest Pumpkin and Sausage Soup	Keto and Dairy-Free Vanilla Custard
24	Keto Cinnamon Coffee	Keto Chinese Pork Stew with Cabbage	Coconut Mahi-Mahi Nuggets	Creamed Fruit Salad
25	Keto Coconut Flake Balls	Keto Harvest Pumpkin and Sausage Soup	Salmon Skewers in Cured Ham	Deliciously Cold Lychee Sorbet
26	Chocolate Banana Smoothie	Garlic Steak Bite Salad with Tarragon Dressing	Stuffed Keto Mushrooms	Oat and Fruit Parfait
27	Smoked Salmon and Poached Eggs on Toast	Cod Loin with Horseradish and Browned Butter	Sweet Garlic Chicken Skewers	Chocolate Mug Muffins
28	Fruit Smoothie	Stuffed Keto Mushrooms	Cilantro Chicken Breasts with Mayo-Avocado Sauce	Chocolate Spread with Hazelnuts

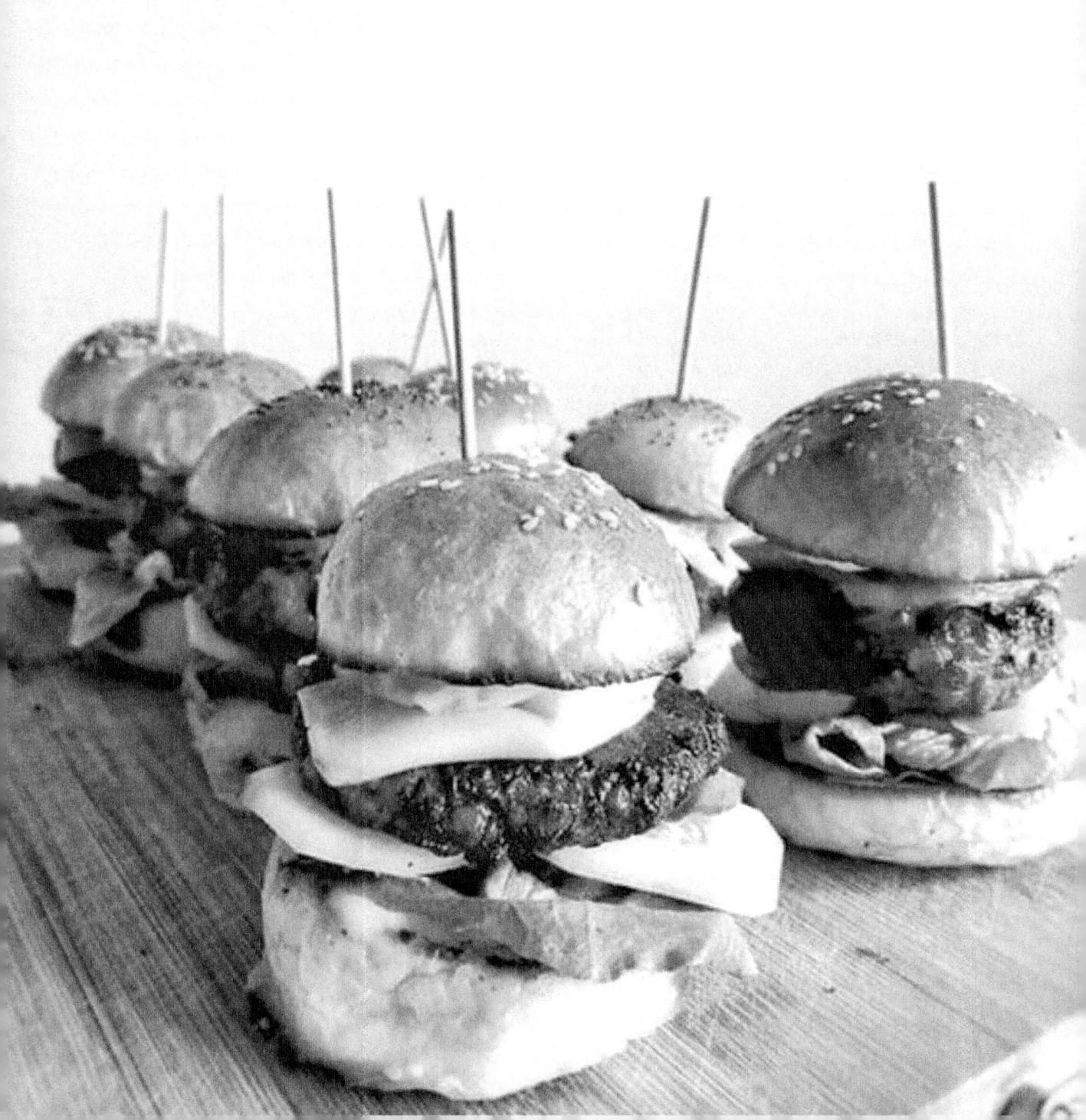

Conclusion

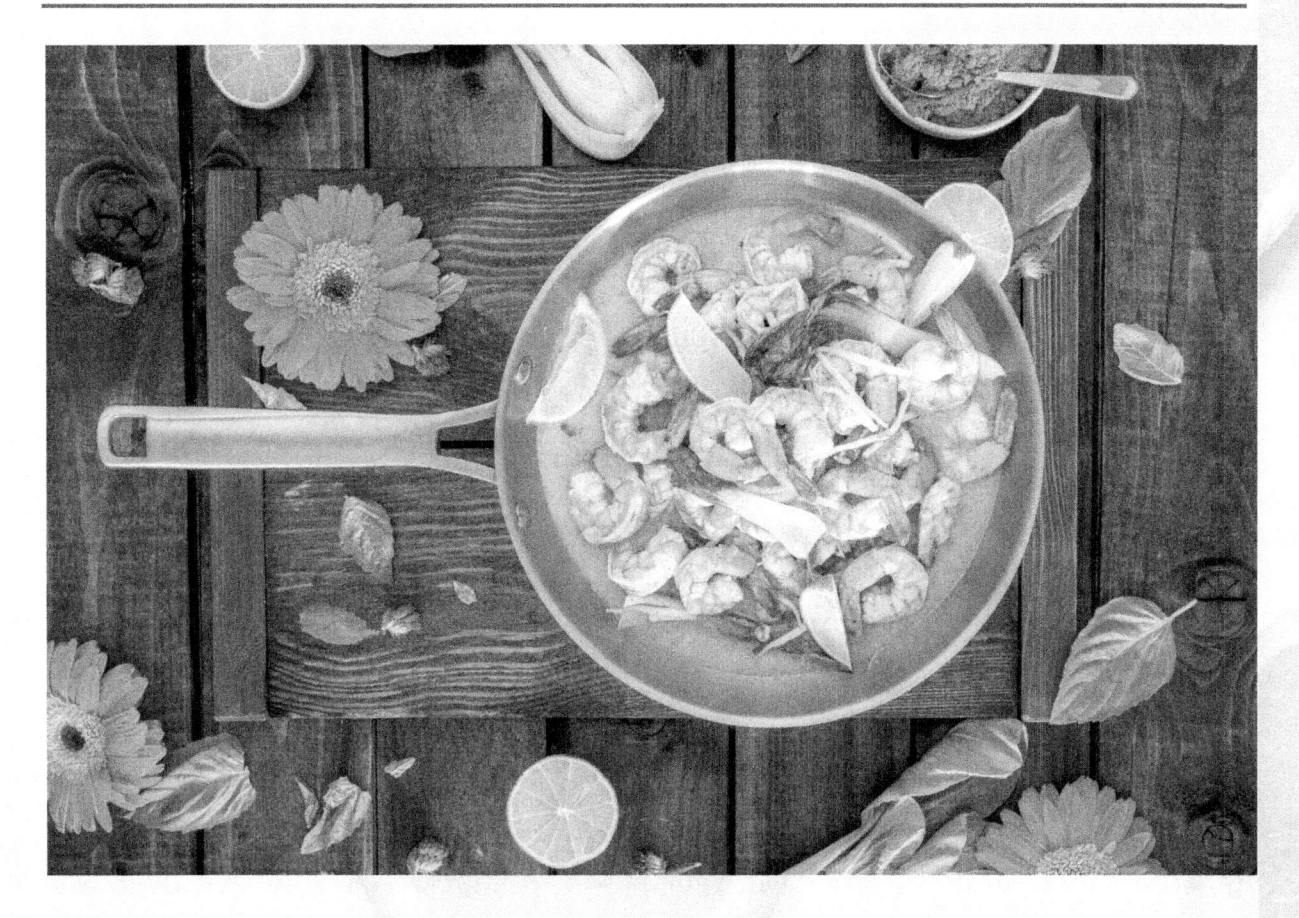

The Keto diet as we have read and emphasized provides for and enables, by minimizing carbohydrates, maximizing the consumption of vegetable and animal fats and making sure to take in the necessary protein, training regularly and resting effectively...to lose weight and to plan for a future of sound psycho-physical health...and why not...even happiness.

In this guide you will find all the information you need to begin this personal hike of yours through the grasslands of nutrition linked to physical training and much-needed restful rest. Considering that all aspects, particularly for adult-mature people, are interconnected and players all together in your long-term success...and also in your failure.

It is quite common practice to face challenging choices such as changing one's habits, putting one's head down, following the food plan to the letter, suffering deprivations passively and hoping for a positive outcome...if you have read the pages so far I hope you have realized that this is not the case...right?

When you are faced with painful, complicated and challenging situations, you should remind yourself of WHY you started. Choices are always bets we make with ourselves first, which is why it is good to emphasize that our mental commitment is paramount in defining our success or defeat.

Dieting begins in our brains, and the most useful results for ourselves will be right in our minds, the most outward and obvious ones in our bodies, to the satisfaction of our egos and the society around us.

Mature adults need to take care of themselves like never before, so if you have never made yourself your top priority, do it now. It is time to adopt healthy habits and stop procrastinating, to do everything in your power to improve mentally and then as a consequence ... physically.

Get our priorities in order, write them down in a journal, check where we are at, train, take care of ourselves, rest and find some peace. These should be the goals for the most important person in our lives, our family members and few friends...US.

As you read carefully you will find all the technical information you need to face this challenge in the best possible way. For an adult-mature beginner to get off on the right foot thus avoiding the yo yo effect...so recurrent and feared by beginners, you need the right holistic approach. A strategy, perseverance and determination.

Figuring out right away what one is up against when implementing such a choice is impossible...the answers will come during the journey...positive or negative.

Moments of crisis should not frighten us; on the contrary, they should stimulate that mental evolution that will help keep us on track, help us be more conscious, respectful and satisfying for our planet, for ourselves and for our species.

I have written other books on these topics...connecting the dots...it is always a good idea to realize what is represented in the full picture, this top-down view allows us to analyze our decisions and continue or change attitude and behavior in the present and future.

Best of luck.

P.S.

Your opinion on the book you just read is very important to me!

My goal is to know how to publish books of better quality in the future and to update and improve existing ones.

So, it would be great reading your feedback. Thank you

Best, Penny Craig

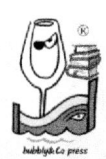

Author Overview

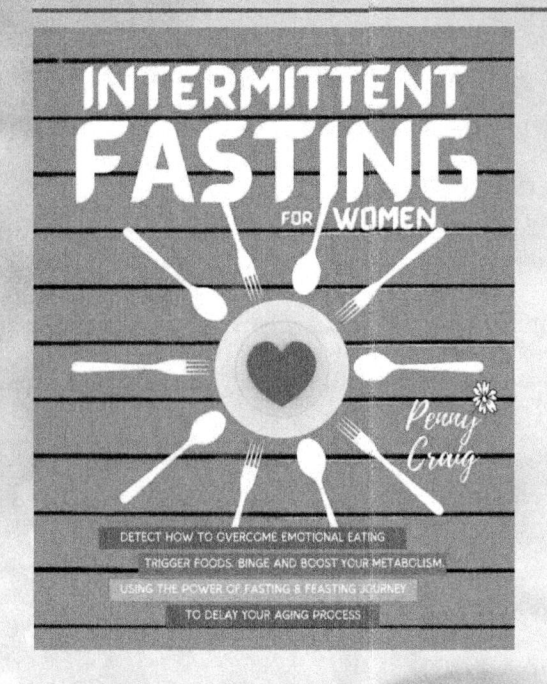

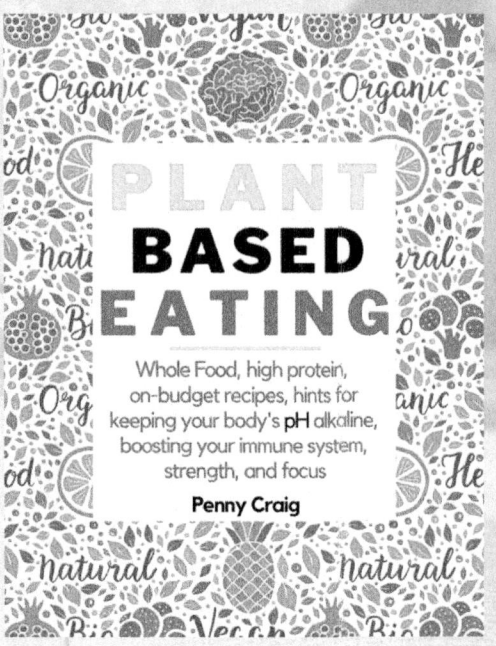

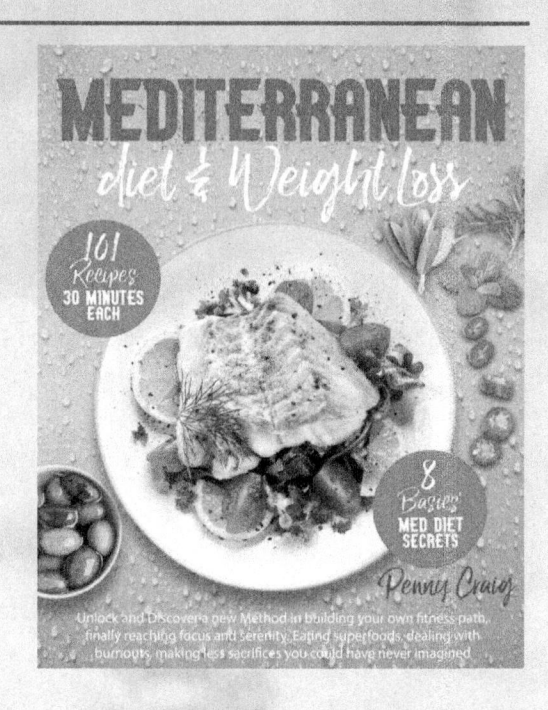

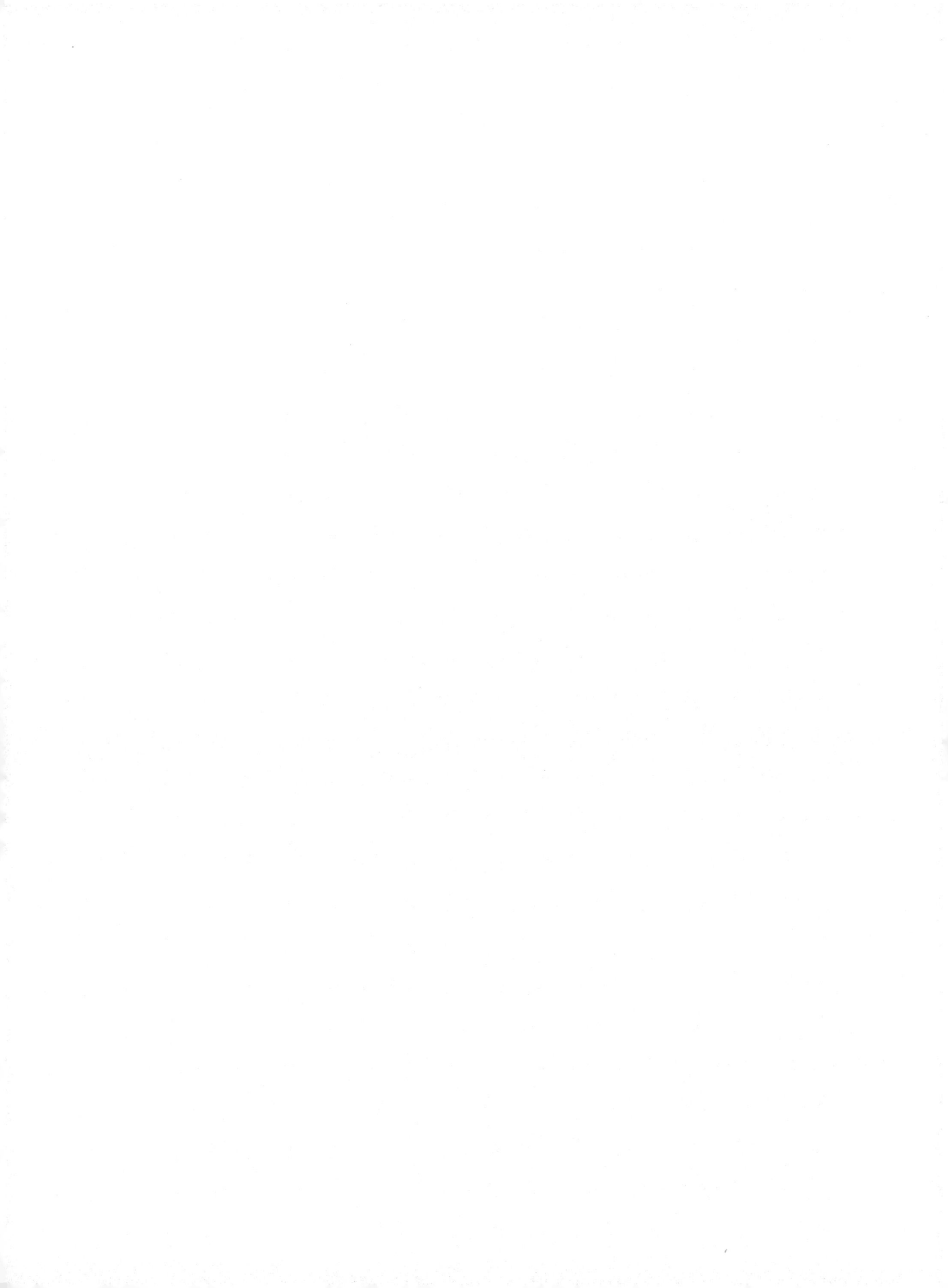

Printed in Great Britain
by Amazon